FERTILE GROUND

Faith Tested.

Truth Revealed.

Destiny Fulfilled.

Stacy Davis Stanton

Wasteland Press
Shelbyville, KY USA
www.wastelandpress.net

Fertile Ground:
Faith Tested. Truth Revealed. Destiny Fulfilled.
By Stacy Davis Stanton

Copyright © 2010 Stacy Davis Stanton
ALL RIGHTS RESERVED

First Printing – May 2010
ISBN: 978-1-60047-443-9

Unless otherwise indicated, all Bible quotations were taken from the King James Version of the Bible.

NO PART OF THIS BOOK MAY BE REPRODUCED IN ANY FORM, BY PHOTOCOPYING OR BY ANY ELECTRONIC OR MECHANICAL MEANS, INCLUDING INFORMATION STORAGE OR RETRIEVAL SYSTEMS, WITHOUT PERMISSION IN WRITING FROM THE COPYRIGHT OWNER/AUTHOR

Printed in the U.S.A.

Acknowledgements

First and foremost, I offer praise and thanksgiving to my Lord and Savior, Jesus Christ for giving me the courage, not only to go through the storm, but to share the testimony. I love, honor, and glorify you in all things.

I offer my sincere gratitude to:

My partner in life, my husband, Barry Jerome Stanton, for his enduring strength and undying support for me and for this project. I love you beyond measure.

Caleb, for being my daily reminder of how awesome God is. You are my precious gift from God, and I am honored to be your mommy.

My mother, Lonnie Davis, for your continuous love and encouragement. Thank you for praying for me when I didn't have the forethought to pray for myself. I love you!

My grandmother, Ms. Madie Wynn, for praying for me, for comforting me, for believing what God would do for me. I love you!

My sister, Yashica, for being a rock, a friend, a confidant, and prayer warrior. I love you!

Stephanie Dixon, a living, breathing example of undying friendship. Thank you for all the times you listened and encouraged me.

Mrs. Sonja Fulcher, for going through the storm with me. You were there every step of the way. I love you for that!

Mrs. Kisha Wesley for the calls, especially on Angel's birthday, the encouraging words, the cards, the faithfulness of your friendship.

Mrs. Alysia Anderson, for never forgetting Angel's birthday, for taking a flight to be with me when I was down, for abiding sisterhood, and for your prayers.

My "big sister by one day," Ms. Toni Dupree, for believing with me. Know that God will bless you with your heart's desires in His time.

Ms. Lorrie Harrison, for the little things you might have thought went unnoticed like taking a flight to be with me or visiting Yashica in the hospital.

My friend, Mrs. Alaina Higgins and my sister-in-law, Mrs. Nicole Brand for calling me every week during my pregnancy with Caleb just to see if everything was okay.

My nieces and nephews who brighten my life – Jayden, Justin, Tionna, Ethan, KaJayla, and Janesha. Auntie loves you so much!

My little brother, Henri, for being such an awesome part of my life.

My godson, Sterling Andrew Higgins, for your loving smile, infectious laughter, and all the joy you've brought me.

Dr. Reginald Robinson and the entire staff of Chatham OB/GYN for your compassion and professionalism. I will never forget you, Sharon, Chiquita, Linda, and Felicia! You guys truly became an extension of my family!

Rev. Dr. Matthew M. Odum, Sr. for teaching me *how* to pray and *how* to exercise my faith and for believing when I found it hard to.

The prayer warriors of Temple of Glory Community Church. There are too many to name, but you know who you are.

Everyone who ever interceded on my behalf with a prayer of expectancy, I am eternally grateful!

Table of Contents

1.	Awake Me From This Nightmare	1
2.	The Perfect Plan	15
3.	Just Another Ordinary Day	18
4.	Take Two	23
5.	Under the Knife-Over the Hurdle	32
6.	Walking Out of the Valley	38
7.	Evidence of Things Not Seen	45
8.	New Assignment-New Calling	57
9.	Turning Point	65
10.	Revelation	71
11.	The Prophecy	77
12.	Faithful is our God	83
13.	The Perfect Pregnancy	91
14.	The Manifestation	97
	Epilogue	104

CHAPTER ONE

Awake Me from This Nightmare

Light as a glaring sun pierces through my transparent shell. As I struggle to gather my facilities, I helplessly reach for the remnants of hope I had for a miracle. What does all this mean? Just minutes after hearing the rhythm of a faint, but sweet heartbeat, I am in receipt of the news that my dream has been ripped from my very being. What is this? Could this really be happening? In voices that sounded as distant as the day is long, I could hear, "15:55! Log the time of birth! 15:55!"

A feeling of joy swept through me as a hurricane on an unsuspecting coast. Was she okay? I knew she was here because I had heard the announcement of the birth time. I needed to know. I just had to know! At that moment, the only feeling of comfort that existed was the stroke of my husband's hand across my perspiring forehead.

This all happened so fast. It was nearly impossible to process. I could not wrap my mind around the devastating words floating about the room like a bird's feather left behind. In my sedation and fragile state of mind, I could only decipher fragments of the message.

"I'm sorry. She was just too small."

The words sounded as though they had been choreographed – a song recorded in a studio and played a million times for diverse audiences. Why couldn't I change the station or turn it off altogether? Did I have to hear this? Would this nightmare soon subside? It was a nightmare, wasn't it? This couldn't really be happening. It just couldn't be. I had named her. We had decided to call her Gabrielle, a name meaning "God is my strength."

She was mine. She had moved about my womb as if trying to find the comfortable spot on the bed. The date for the shower had been set. I was ready to hold her and had even settled into the reality of sleepless nights and years of responsibility. She was the most beautiful part of me. She was the ultimate expression of the love my husband and I shared. I had waited with great anticipation for her arrival. It was to be a time of rejoicing for my family.

What had gone wrong? The date was March 3, 2004, and this nightmare had begun just nine days prior when I reported to my doctor's office for a routine ultrasound. I am of the opinion that this is one of the best doctors of obstetrics and gynecology in the Savannah area, not because he has mastered some magical technique, but because he seems to genuinely care about the welfare of his patients. It was his compassion and attentiveness that helped to soften the blow of this ordeal.

To be quite honest, I was caught off guard. I mean, I know I had not had a perfect pregnancy, but this somehow seemed different. So, how was it that I ended up in this desolate place once again? How on earth could this be happening?

I learned of this pregnancy in October 2003. My husband, Jerome, and I were residing with my mother while our home was under construction. In this transitional period in my life, I had become completely consumed by life's mundane daily routine. My days were largely spent discussing details of the house, working, and spending time with my younger brother and nephew.

It was no secret that I strongly desired to become a mother. Anyone who knew me knew that having children was a key part of my *perfect plan*. My desire was such that some would assume that I was oblivious to the fact that having and raising children required a great deal of intestinal fortitude. Yes, I was fully aware of the challenges involved in the rearing of children. My focus, however, was never really on the *challenges* of parenting, but rather the *rewards* of doing so. I often thought of the many ways I could use my own life experiences, good and bad, to help shape this young person into a strong, spiritually grounded, and productive adult.

It was my belief that I was divinely appointed to become a mother. I believed it was God's will that I have children of my own. I further believed the roles I had played in the lives of so many children, including my 4-year-old nephew and 6-year-old brother had adequately prepared me to embrace a child of my own.

Now, if this were true, and if it were that simple, the most recent chain of events did not add up. If it was indeed God's perfect will for me to become a mother, why would He deny me that very thing? Is that what He had done? It certainly seemed that way. It just didn't add up.

The news of this pregnancy was bittersweet for me. Having suffered two miscarriages, I was what some would refer to as cautiously optimistic. My husband and I wanted to be parents, and now it was happening for us. The excitement of purchasing our first home was compounded by the news of my third pregnancy.

It never occurred to us that this would not be a successful pregnancy. Maybe we were careless and a bit naïve to discount the possibility, or maybe we were just so certain this could not happen. After all, should this pregnancy fail, it would be the third loss for us. That didn't happen to people, did it? Furthermore, it didn't happen to people who believed and stood firmly on the word of God. It was around this premise that we built our false sense of security.

I exercised due diligence in attending doctor's appointments. Given my history, my doctor ordered more frequent visits and ultrasounds to ensure any potential problems would be caught early. In an attempt to explain what could have possibly caused my previous miscarriages, he told me of a condition called cervical incompetence. This was a condition in which the cervix, the opening to the uterus, becomes structurally weak and could open up without warning. For a woman suffering from cervical incompetence, there is often no pain associated with miscarriages. The cervix simply opens up, and the pregnancy is aborted.

Although I had experienced severe pain during both miscarriages, not characteristic of cervical incompetence, my doctor offered to stitch my cervix closed as a precaution. The stitch, known as a cervical cerclage, would be placed during an outpatient procedure and would hold the cervix closed, preventing preterm labor. I was advised that the procedure carried such risks as rupture of the amniotic sack, which could lead to preterm labor. I was also advised that this procedure was not usually done prior to 12 weeks' gestation.

Armed with all the information I believed I needed, I scheduled my surgery for the first week in December. For some reason, I was not nervous. I viewed this as a measure of precaution and failed to give much consideration to the possibility that my pregnancy might be in trouble.

Although this was normally an outpatient procedure, Dr. Robinson wanted me to spend one night in the hospital after the surgery for observation. The cerclage was successfully placed on December 1, 2003. Dr. Robinson advised me that my cervix was short and that its length presented some challenges in placing the cerclage. Despite the challenges, my cervix was stitched closed. After a week of resting and recovering at home, I was back to my normal routine – work, spending time with family, having random thoughts about the baby, and just going about life as if nothing was wrong. After all, nothing *was* wrong. I was gradually overcoming the affects of morning sickness and was even adjusting to my growing belly. I was pregnant, and it was exciting!

After two miscarriages, I was well on my way to joining the elite club of women that now included several of my friends. God is awesome, and He was truly showing favor. My husband and I had closed on our home in late November and were thinking of ways to decorate the nursery. During an ultrasound in January 2004, we received the exciting news that I was carrying a little girl. My sister, Yashica, had settled on May 15th as the date for the baby shower. What an exciting time! Our perfect plan was coming together. In all the excitement, I never asked God to reveal His perfect will to us. I just assumed we were walking in it.

It was a beautiful Monday morning, and I was rushing through the employee entrance at the Georgia Department of Labor. As my supervisor walked past my cubicle, I gently tapped him on the shoulder.

"Mr. Alston, don't forget I have a doctor's appointment this morning."

He smiled and nodded as if to say, "I'm sure everything's going to be just fine."

I smiled as if I believed just that. I was at work for approximately one hour before it was time to leave. When you're pregnant, each doctor's appointment is an exciting adventure. With my cervical cerclage securely in place, I was certain that this journey would have a happy ending.

I grabbed my purse and keys and headed for the door. As I walked through the parking lot to my car, I wondered what we would do to celebrate my mother's birthday, which happened to be the next day, February 24th. Maybe we could do dinner. I was sure that once I spoke with my sister, we would figure something out. It was such a beautiful day, and I couldn't help thinking how awesome God was. I was so grateful to be receiving such wonderful blessings. It never occurred to me that I was not as spiritually connected as I should be. I was definitely experiencing spiritual growth, but my faith had not been tested to the degree it soon would be. So, how strong was my desire to get closer to God? I would soon have to search the very depths of myself to truly find the answer to that question.

When I arrived at the doctor's office, I was reminded that I would have an ultrasound but would not actually meet with my doctor until Wednesday. "Great!" I thought. Today would be pretty uneventful – just a routine ultrasound. The further I progressed in my pregnancy, the more excited I became. I was now one day short of reaching 23 weeks' gestation. Every doctor's appointment, every ultrasound, and even every little change I noticed in my body excited me beyond description. I was especially elated to learn I was carrying a little girl – a beautiful little girl.

I settled into a room that had become all too familiar to me – the ultrasound room. As the ultrasound technician entered the room, she was met by my vehement excitement. She glanced at my chart and gave me a look that seemed to say, "I can see you're excited, so let's get this show on the road." The lights had been dimmed, and I slowly positioned myself on the examination table. As previously instructed, I reminded the technician that I had a cerclage in place.

The room was dark; I was undressed from the waist down; and the equipment was all set. My ultrasound was about to begin. "Ahhh, there's my little girl," I thought, "and look at that heart go!" I wondered what she would be like. Would she inherit my personality or that of her father's? Would she be into sports? Would she be a girly girl? My heart seemed to skip a beat at the mere thought of giving birth to this beautiful little angel. After examining the baby's heartbeat and movement, the technician reminded me that I would also be undergoing a transvaginal ultrasound, something I enjoyed almost as much as I enjoyed morning sickness and heartburn. Within minutes, my routine ultrasound was over.

"Okay, go ahead and get dressed, and I'll be back in just a moment." The ultrasound technician never looked up at me.

I hopped off the table and began putting myself back together. Just as I was about to put my shoes on, I paused. At that very moment, I was hit with the overwhelming feeling that something might be wrong. I couldn't put my finger on it, but I couldn't shake the feeling. The ultrasound technician had asked me to get dressed and wait for her to return. Normally when I underwent a routine ultrasound, I was given a few pictures and reminded of my next appointment. The technician had never asked me to wait for her to return.

My heart began racing as I imagined all the things that could possibly be going wrong. My palms began to sweat, and without even realizing it, I grabbed my abdominal area. I spoke softly to the vibrant little baby I had just seen on the ultrasound.

"Are you okay in there? Mommy won't let anything happen to you."

My conversation with my baby was interrupted by the return of the ultrasound technician who informed me that Dr. Robinson would be in to see me in just a few moments. At this point, I knew that something was wrong. I was not supposed to see Dr. Robinson for another two days. I continued to talk to my baby – and to myself – in an attempt to shake this menacing anxiety I was experiencing.

Somewhere between my heart palpitations and my failed attempt at reassurance, Dr. Robinson walked into the room. At first glance, he appeared a little frazzled. I followed his every move with my eyes.

"Do you want the good news or the bad news?"

"What's going on?"

"Well, the good news is that everything is still intact. The bad news is that if we don't do something quickly, that could change."

"So, what do we need to do?" I asked, my voice trembling.

"I'm putting you in the hospital for a long time."

"How long?" I asked slowly.

"Until after the baby is born."

I did not respond to Dr. Robinson's last comment. I just sat on the table and stared at him as if I was waiting for a punch line. I started thinking how serious this must have been. If I was being ordered to spend the duration of my pregnancy in the hospital, something must have been terribly wrong. So many thoughts raced through my mind, but nothing came out of my mouth. It was like I could not conjure up the courage to inquire further. So, I just sat there.

Dr. Robinson looked at me like a father who was telling a child her pet had died. He was very serious. Very calculated. While he wanted to demonstrate compassion, he wanted to tell me the unadulterated truth. He needed for me to understand that my pregnancy was in trouble. He slowly continued with his explanation.

"Your cervix appears to be opening up. Too much pressure on your cervix could send you into preterm labor very quickly. Even with the cerclage in place, there could be a rupture of membranes."

This was such strange news to me because I had not experienced any pain or discomfort. I would have never guessed that something like this was happening. I didn't care how it had happened or when it began. All I wanted to know was how to rectify it. At this point, I was just a mother trying to save her child. I was fighting back tears as I tried to process everything that had been conveyed to me.

"So, when do I need to report to the hospital?"

"I will be back with some paperwork for you. Take a moment to contact your family and your employer and report to Memorial Health as soon as possible."

"Okay, I will."

Just as Dr. Robinson turned to walk out of the room, I released the tears I had been fighting back so hard. It was February 23, 2004, and my baby girl was not due until June 24th. As I sat in that small ultrasound room, I felt so helpless. No one had accompanied me to this appointment because it was only supposed to be a routine ultrasound. There was not to be much fanfare. How did I go from that to the news that I would be spending the duration of my pregnancy in the hospital? Even more grueling than the thought of the hospital stay was the harsh reality that my pregnancy was in serious trouble.

After breaking the news to Jerome and my employer, I retreated to my mother's house. She accompanied me to get some items packed, and we met Jerome at the hospital. I was officially admitted at approximately 3:30pm and was immediately given muscle relaxers in an effort to prevent contractions.

There I was, in the hospital, surrounded by people who were making honest attempts to assure me that things were not as bad as I believed them to be. It didn't take a rocket scientist to realize that my doctor would not have taken such a drastic measure if nothing had been wrong. It was glaringly obvious that there was cause for concern, alarm even.

No matter what this picture was starting to look like, I made the conscious decision to turn to the one thing I knew would get me through this – my faith. I knew I served a God who would never leave or forsake me. I was on the verge of a journey religion could not help me with. I needed something more binding. I needed a close, personal relationship with God. I needed the type of relationship that would sustain me when the forecast was bleak. I needed to feel God's presence, and I needed it right away!

After two long, monotonous days in the hospital, I met with my doctor, who had enlisted the assistance of a team of perinatologists. One member of the team had met with me during my second day in the hospital and had explained to me that my cervix, which was short, was showing signs of beaking, or funneling. Of course, I had no idea what this meant, but I knew it was not something that was *supposed* to be happening. It was explained to me that uterine pressure was causing the cervix to gradually open from the top and to take on a Y-shape. If this continued, I could experience a sudden rupture of membranes.

At the advice of the prenatal team, Dr. Robinson reluctantly decided to release me from the hospital with the express stipulation that I be placed on strict bed rest. Realizing how mundane a hospital stay would be, I readily embraced the alternative. I thought being in the comfort of my own home would somehow take my mind off the glaring fact that my pregnancy was in serious trouble. Dr. Robinson requested that I return to his office the following Monday for a follow-up.

"Well, in case you're wondering, I'm putting you back in the hospital."

My eyes followed Dr. Robinson as he paced about the small examination room. I could not even bring myself to ask what was wrong. This situation was becoming much larger than me. Although I did not ask the question out loud, he went on to explain to me that my cervix was still enduring too much pressure and that it was trying to open up. The plan would be to admit me to the hospital, monitor any contractions I might have, and keep me on bed rest except for restroom breaks. Dr. Robinson even went so far as to request that I report to the hospital immediately, unlike I had done the previous week.

I was amazed at how my season of immense joy had given way to a time of fear, anxiety, and most of all, uncertainty. No matter how sincere the efforts to comfort me, my dubious state of mind would no longer allow me to sink into this cozy, but false sense of security. I may have been a day late and a dollar short, but I now had my guard up. Cumbersome was the task of preparing for the worst possible outcome, but it was something I had to do. Throughout my pregnancy and even in these terrifying hours, my husband remained the eternal optimist. Because I had experienced some noticeable growth in my spiritual walk, I allowed myself to believe that by praying and declaring that this pregnancy would be a successful one, I had secured a positive outcome. However, there was one pertinent piece missing from the puzzle – seeking the perfect will of God. It's funny how we can look back and realize we weren't quite where we needed to be spiritually at times when we thought we had it all figured out.

So caught up in my master plan of motherhood, I failed to ask God to direct me according to His plan. I did the opposite of what God's word commands us to do. I leaned on my own understanding. To that end, I refused to accept what was beginning to seem like the inevitable.

March 2, 2004 was a day of little fanfare. As I lay in my hospital bed with an IV and several monitors connected to me, the medical staff came and went in their usual haste, checking vital signs and ensuring I was comfortable. It wasn't until that evening, around the time shifts were changing, that I noticed that something was just not right. I began to experience cramps of moderate intensity. What concerned me was that they came and went at a slow, but steady paste, almost like contractions.

When Dr. Robinson entered the room to check on me, he checked the monitor and noticed that I had registered several contractions. Although the contractions had not been severe, they did show on the monitor. Dr. Robinson stressed the importance of staying in bed unless I was going to the restroom. He did not want me getting out of bed for *any* other reason. He ordered the nursing staff to continue administering magnesium sulfate in an effort to halt my impending labor.

Notwithstanding the contractions, my night was pretty uneventful. My sister stopped by with snacks and magazines to aid in making me more comfortable. My mother had informed me that a young lady with whom she worked had delivered her baby earlier that day at 24 weeks' gestation. Although born prematurely and very small, the baby was holding on. Having just reached my 24th week, I was reassured by hearing this. I thought that even if my little girl was born early, she would be okay. I thought...

After my sister left, and Jerome and I settled in for the night, I had trouble sleeping. I was still having mild menstrual-like cramps, and I was also very anxious. I couldn't stop thinking about the fact that I had already begun having contractions, and my baby wasn't due for another 16 weeks. I looked over at Jerome, who somehow managed to drift off to sleep on that uncomfortable cot. He looked so peaceful. He worried so much about me and our baby, but he went to great lengths to exude strength. Although I knew he couldn't be too comfortable on that cot, I knew he needed whatever rest he was able to get. I just watched him sleep until I managed to drift off myself.

On the morning of March 3rd, I made a concerted effort to subdue my fears and embrace the day with optimism. However, I had this feeling that something just would not be right about this day. I was anxious. I was crying every few minutes. I was still having mild contractions even though I was still receiving magnesium sulfate. Because of the risks associated with magnesium sulfate, I could only be given a certain dosage. If the dosage I had been given was not halting my contractions, there may not have been any other recourse to curtail labor. As I became more listless, the contractions became a little more intense.

My nurse followed my activity very closely that morning. During one of her many visits to my room, she did something extremely unorthodox. She asked if she could pray with me. She explained that she didn't always do this, but she felt that I was a spiritual person. On the other hand, I was usually very guarded about who I allowed to pray with me and for me, but I had a good feeling about this young lady. We joined hands and both said a prayer. She looked me square in the eye and told me to remember that God does not do anything without good reason and that He was with me in that room.

I was trying so hard to pull myself together because I was looking forward to having lunch with my friends, Sonja and Nicole who had made plans to spend their lunch break with me. Something in my spirit was telling me that they probably shouldn't come on that particular day. Even though I had prayed, I began to feel very uneasy, very anxious. It was the same feeling I had been trying to suppress since the previous night. I couldn't shake it, but I knew something wasn't right. In fact, when Sonja called to discuss lunch plans, I told her I thought maybe she and Nicole should come on another day because I wasn't feeling well. What I didn't tell Sonja was that it was more than that. It was not as simple as me not feeling well. I was fearful that something was about to happen. When I told Sonja not to come to the hospital, I almost felt that I was protecting her from something. It kind of reminded me of the way my father refused to allow anyone to ride in the car with him just days before he died in a car accident.

Even though I had already prayed, I prayed again. As my feelings of anxiety coalesced with the fact that I was having contractions, I began to mentally prepare myself for a tragic outcome. It was as if my mind was preparing me for the worst, but my heart was still in the fight for a positive outcome. How could it not be? This was my baby girl! How could my heart not tell me to fight to save her?

As I sat quietly on my bed, staring at nothing in particular, a small, unassuming woman walked into my room.

"Hello?" I lifted my head to see who was walking in.

"Hi, how are you, Stacy?"

"I-I'm okay," I said, still very confused as to who this woman was.

"I know you don't know me," she continued, "but I work with your sister. She told me a little bit about what you have been going through. My name is Ms. Louise."

Yashica had told me of a woman on her job who was very spiritual and who often encouraged her.

"Oh, yes," I responded, "My sister has mentioned you before."

"I hope you don't mind me stopping by. I won't stay long. I just wanted to give you something."

"Oh, sure. That's okay. I don't mind."

At that moment, Ms. Louise pulled out a beautiful purple book titled *Speak to My Heart, God*. She slowly handed the book to me and told me that she was praying for me. She told me that she wouldn't stay long because she knew I needed my rest.

"Thank you for stopping by and for your prayers."

Ms. Louise rested her hand on my shoulder and nodded. She told me to get some rest, and as quickly as she had entered my room, she left. I just sat looking in the direction of the door for a few moments. Then I slowly turned my attention back to the book. I opened it up, and there was a passage of scripture that had encouraged me many times before. The passage was Romans 8:28, which reads:

And we know that all things work together for good to them that love God, to them who are the called according to His purpose.

As the day progressed, I could not fully prepare myself for what *all things* would entail. At approximately 1:30pm, I began to notice a marked increase in the intensity and frequency of my contractions. Although the pain was starting to intensify, and I was feeling extremely lethargic, I managed to get myself up to go to the restroom. During this restroom visit, I noticed something unnerving. I noticed a spot of blood about the size of a quarter. I immediately notified my nurse who placed a call to Dr. Robinson. She returned and informed me that Dr. Robinson did not want me out of the bed for any reason, not even to go to the restroom. As my nurse monitored my contractions, she noticed they were about six minutes apart. She looked at me with a very sympathetic expression on her face.

"Mrs. Stanton, I don't think we are going to be able to stop your labor because your contractions are getting closer together."

"But even if we can't stop the labor, we should be okay, right? I can hear the baby's heartbeat."

"I'm going to tell Dr. Robinson about your contractions. He will probably want to come and check you out for himself."

I noticed how my nurse avoided my question. I knew that all signs pointed to trouble, but I was holding on to the sound of my baby's heartbeat with everything I had. It was the only thing that soothed me at that moment. When Yashica called to check on me, I explained to her that I was in labor and that the baby might be coming that day. She left work and rushed to the hospital.

As Yashica and I sat there, I was beginning to feel so exhausted and so weary. The only thing keeping me awake was the pain of my contractions. It was like no pain I had experienced before. My sister sat there, rubbing my head as medical staff rushed in and out of my room. As I lay there, I began to bleed profusely. Too weak to do so myself, I asked Yashica to look under the covers to assess the situation. As she pulled the sheets back, there was bright, red blood all over the bed. She made a frantic call to my nurse, who informed me that Dr. Robinson was on the way. After getting the nurse, Yashica made two very difficult phone calls – one to Jerome and one to my mother. They both left their jobs and rushed to the hospital.

By the time Dr. Robinson arrived, my contractions were less than three minutes apart and I was hemorrhaging at an alarming rate. Dr. Robinson informed me that he was going to deliver the baby by cesarean section. With a melancholy expression on his face, he explained to me that it was too soon for the baby but that we had no choice but to deliver her.

I lay there helpless, in pain, and hemorrhaging as the medical staff began to prep me for surgery. Even though I was barely coherent, I could see Dr. Robinson beckon my family to come into the hallway. I would not learn until later what he was sharing with them.

Everything was happening so fast. Dr. Robinson wanted to get the baby delivered before I lost too much blood. I was so weak that I was barely aware of the conversations going on all around me. I don't remember much about that moment, but I do remember being moved from my bed, being placed on a gurney, and being wheeled to the operating room. I vaguely remember receiving an epidural. Everything else was very fuzzy until…

I heard the announcement that my daughter had been born at 3:55pm. Just like that, she had made her entry into the world. She was born with a strong heartbeat and no chance of survival. Attempts to insert tubes to help her breathe were unsuccessful. It wasn't a nightmare as I had hoped. It was real. Jerome and I named her Angel Faithe Stanton, not Gabrielle as was the original plan.

For nine days, I had been on an emotional, mental, and physical roller coaster ride. I was having so much trouble processing the fact that at 24 weeks, I had suffered the loss of my third confirmed pregnancy. I did not get it. I wanted to ask God why because it wasn't supposed to go this way.

Faced with many difficult choices, Jerome and I opted for direct cremation of our daughter. I am usually an amazingly strong person, but I had been reduced to a shell of a mother who would have died to save her child. After Angel's birth and demise, I was informed that Dr. Robinson had called my family out into the hallway to explain to them that the choice had come down to trying to save me or my baby. Because I had lost so much blood, he felt I would not live through the night had the baby not been delivered when she was. As a mother, the choice I would have made might have been different from the one that was actually made. I would have given my life in a second to save that little girl, or even to give her a little more time. For the first time, I truly knew what motherhood felt like.

This day, this experience, and this point in time represented a defining moment in my faith walk. It was time for me to believe or let my dream die. It was time for me to prove to God that my desire to please Him and to live for Him far exceeded my desire for anything else. The time had come. It remained to be seen how I would handle it.

CHAPTER TWO

The Perfect Plan

To understand the gravity of losing Angel the way we did, it became necessary for Jerome and I to reflect on the well-laid plan we thought to be full-proof. In the days and weeks following Angel's demise, I began the arduous task of examining myself. Amidst feelings of guilt and shame, I had to find one reason to hold on to my dream of becoming a mother. Whatever the reason, it had to be compelling enough to get me through the tough days. I had no idea just how many *tough days* were ahead of me.

When you combine guilt, shame, and grief, you have a suicidal combination of emotions. While the idea of suicide seems so extreme, it is a sad reality for so many. For me, it took constant prayer and a willingness to become naked before God to deter any thoughts that I might not want to go on. What you need to truly understand is that the line between committing suicide and making the decision to continue living is very thin. It can sometimes be as simple as believing and trusting God's word or not doing so.

When I really think about it, though, I realize that I never wanted to die during this process. I just wanted my babies to live. Was that too much to ask? Was God really listening? What had I done in my life that was so terrible that I had to pay with my children's lives? I had now begun the prodigious task of examining this situation from all angles and seeking a deeper answer to the resounding question, "Why?"

After our marriage in August 2000, Jerome and I set the foundation for our perfect plan. We knew there were certain goals we wished to attain before entering the ever-changing world of parenthood. Among those was my completion of graduate school. I knew being a new mother would present challenges as I sought my degree. We also desired to become homeowners prior to expanding our family.

The old adage tells us that hindsight is 20/20. That statement couldn't be more true, especially as it pertained to our particular situation. There we were, a young couple with so much promise. We made the erroneous assumption that we could map out every detail of our lives and time all major events just the way we wanted. It's really quite amazing to think that although we were attending church regularly and growing spiritually, we never took the time to ask God to reveal His plan for our lives. Not realizing that God would use this experience to build our faith walk, we focused primarily on what we wanted and when we wanted it.

The plan we laid for ourselves was really quite simple. Simple, but perfect. It was, by all accounts, representative of the American dream. God has an awesome way of manifesting in you His purpose, and His purpose is not founded on the American dream. It is rooted in His word. While we were going about our lives and waiting for our perfect plan to unfold, we missed what God was doing. We missed His perfect will for our lives, at least until much later.

The situation we experienced often reminds me of that quick trip to the supermarket to pick up milk for breakfast. You leave the house. Moments later, you receive a phone call from someone asking you to pick up a few more items. Then you remember that you need cleaning supplies, so you stop by the nearest Family Dollar. When you finally start home, you realize you've forgotten something and turn around. What began as a 15-minute trip to the store has now taken more than an hour. We began trying to have a baby in 2002, and our *quick trip* to parenthood was not supposed to take more than one year. In God's infinite wisdom, He allowed our *quick trip* to take five years. Without warning, our journey went down a path we never saw coming.

What we faced would have broken many marriages, but somehow we came to realize that God had a purpose in what He was allowing to happen. We could not completely wrap our minds around it at the time, but we knew there had to be a purpose. After all, we did not serve a God of pain and desolation. While we were in the storm, His purpose seemed so unclear to us. We just could not understand what reason God would have for the devastation we faced. We would come to better understand God's plan in due time. We would eventually realize what He required of us. Most importantly, we would come to realize that *our* plan does not always line up with *His* plan.

CHAPTER THREE

Just Another Ordinary Day

Once we set our perfect plan in motion, we saw no reason to give any substantial thought to it on a frequent basis. We would just let things take their natural course. In July 2002, I took the only major step I would take to ensure the outcome we desired. I removed oral contraceptives from my daily regimen. Once that was done, I went on with life with little thought to when, or even if, I would become pregnant. The days, weeks, and months began to pass. As far as we were concerned, our journey to parenthood had officially begun. It was just a matter of time.

I often found myself becoming excited at the mere thought of a little person looking into my eyes and depending on me for everything. I could not imagine many responsibilities rendering the same gratification as motherhood. I could hardly wait! I would even find myself working a baby into my current routine, which, by all accounts, was pretty mundane. I spent much of my time going to work, attending church, enjoying time with my family, and exercising with Jerome. There wasn't much fanfare, but I was happy. I was genuinely happy.

It had been several months since I completed graduate school. I often chuckled when thinking back to the response I had given when asked the question of when we planned on starting a family. Without hesitation, I gave what now seems like such an arrogant response.

"I have to give birth to this degree before having any children."

Just who did I think I was? Was I even considering God's purpose for my life? Did I think I could just develop and implement the perfect plan and expect God to follow suit? In retrospect, I realize that I clearly had it all wrong. Boy, was God about to show me just *how* wrong.

The pain of losing Angel was compounded by the fact that we had tasted the unsavory zest of grief and loss in the months prior. It all began on an ordinary day in October 2002. Around the 8th day of October, I began my menstrual cycle. There was nothing particularly unusual about that except the fact that it was much lighter and much shorter than normal. I wrote this change off as my body still adjusting to not taking oral contraceptives. No harm, no foul. Approximately eight days later, however, things took a rather peculiar turn.

On October 16, 2002, I reported to my job at the Georgia Department of Labor feeling fine. In fact, the day was not unlike any other routine day at work. I had a group of clients scheduled for aptitude assessments, so my day began with me organizing materials and setting up the classroom. Approximately 15 minutes before the assessments were to begin, I began to feel sharp pains in my lower back and abdomen. My initial response was to ignore the pain and assume it would eventually subside. After all, I was in perfect health, and there was no cause for alarm. The female body was not without the occasional mysterious pain.

My attempts to ignore the pain were unsuccessful. In fact, I began to alternate between trying to ignore the pain and trying to hide the fact that I was in pain at all. I approached my friend, Sonja, and told her what I was experiencing. She posed the question any woman probably would have under the circumstances.

"Do you think your cycle is about to start?"

"No, that was last week."

"Then maybe it's just gas."

As we shared a brief laugh over her "gas" comment, I experienced another sharp pain. It was as if someone pierced a knife through my lower abdomen and allowed it to exit through my back. Even if I had not had what I thought to be a menstrual cycle a week prior, I would not have to be a rocket scientist to know this was no average menstrual cramp. Be that as it may, I continued with the task at hand.

Having assembled my group, I was going over instructions for the assessment when it happened. I was standing in front of a group of approximately 15 clients when the strangest, most frightening thing happened. There was intense pain, followed by an abrupt release of fluid. I had never been pregnant, but I imagined that what I had just experienced was analogous to what mothers know as "breaking of water."

There was no right way to handle this, so trying as best I could to appear as if nothing was wrong, I excused myself from the room. After securing someone to sit in with my group, I anxiously retreated to the ladies' room, where it became apparent that it was time to call my doctor. The fluid I had spoken of turned out to be blood.

"Oh my God! What's happening to me?" My mind raced, and I thought about the menstrual cycle I had had the previous week. The experience was frightening and unsettling, to say the least. I had experienced my first menstrual cycle at the age of 12, and in nearly 18 years, I had never had a missed or irregular cycle. That fact alone made this ordeal extremely alarming. It was completely atypical for my body.

As I reached for the phone, my palms were full of sweat. I had only had one routine pap smear with Dr. Robinson, but he was no stranger to my family. My sister had spoken highly of him during her pregnancy, but it was not until January 2000 that I actually met Dr. Robinson. He was delivering my nephew, Jayden. Having attempted a vaginal birth, Yashica had to deliver Jayden via cesarean section due to complications that arose during labor. Throughout the ordeal, Dr. Robinson was extremely thorough and attentive.

Prior to meeting Dr. Robinson, I counted myself among those women who preferred to be cared for by female gynecologists. Having witnessed Dr. Robinson's commiserative spirit, however, I decided to enlist his services. His unique combination of professionalism, candor, and compassion would be paramount for the journey Jerome and I were about to embark on.

When the receptionist answered the phone, I explained the details of what had transpired at work. She placed me on hold for a brief period, maybe 30 seconds.

"Mrs. Stanton, we're going to have to ask you to come in immediately."

"Okay, I'm on my way."

I alerted my supervisor and my friend, Sonja, and headed for the door. As I pulled out of the parking lot, I phoned Jerome to explain everything to him. I told him that I would be going home to clean myself up before heading to the doctor. My next call was to my mother, who agreed that the events of the morning had been very strange. She asked that I call her as soon as I found out something from the doctor. Most women know their bodies and know when they are veering off course. This was definitely the case for me. I was not sure *what* the problem was, but I knew there was one.

On my way to the doctor's office, still bleeding and cramping immensely, I called Jerome. For the first time that morning, I said out loud what I was feeling.

"Baby, I'm scared."

"I know," he responded with a voice of reassurance, "I'll meet you there."

Upon arriving at the doctor's office, I went through the standard triage procedures that included a pregnancy test, blood pressure check, and weight check. I was quickly placed in an examination room and told that I would probably be seeing the nurse practitioner. As I waited, I paced the floor. The pain had become so intense that I could not sit. It hurt to sit. It hurt to stand. As I walked about the room in excruciating pain, the nurse practitioner walked in.

"Hi, Mrs. Stanton, are you okay?"

"I don't think I've ever been in this much pain."

"So, it says here that your last menstrual period was last week."

"Yes, or so I thought," I responded, still holding my abdominal area.

"Describe your last menstrual period to me."

"It was very light and only lasted about three days."

"Well," the nurse practitioner said in a sing-songy voice, "Your pregnancy test came back positive."

"It did?" I asked in utter amazement. This was the absolute *last* thing I expected to hear.

"Yes, so now we need to get you into the ultrasound room so we can see if we have a viable pregnancy. That will determine the next step."

I had never been pregnant before, but I did not have to be an expert to know that this was not normal. If my pregnancy was viable, I should not have been bleeding and experiencing this terrible pain. What I was experiencing was in no way consistent with a healthy pregnancy.

The walls of the ultrasound room seemed to be closing in on me as I waited for Dr. Robinson. After what seemed like an eternity, he walked in accompanied by a nurse and the nurse practitioner. He glanced at my chart before speaking.

"This is your first pregnancy, isn't it?"

"Yes," I said, my voice trembling.

"Well, let's see what we have."

He covered my abdominal area with gel and proceeded with the ultrasound. The four of us looked directly at the monitor. None of us saw what we were looking for, an amniotic sac. Before Dr. Robinson uttered a word, it had become painfully obvious what was happening to me. Dr. Robinson described what I was experiencing as a spontaneous abortion. There could be a number of possible explanations. He explained to me that a miscarriage this early in pregnancy could be the body's way of expelling an embryo that isn't developing normally. That was quite a bit to digest.

There I was miscarrying the baby I did not even know I had conceived. Wow! I stared at Dr. Robinson with a somewhat blank expression. I was flooded with random thoughts, and I had so many questions. Had I known about this pregnancy, was there something I could have done to prevent this? Was I on my feet too much at work? What was the explanation for what I thought to be a menstrual cycle the week before?

According to Dr. Robinson, what I had experienced the previous week was likely implantation. He also assured me that miscarriages this early on are not usually preventable. He went on to explain that many women who experience miscarriages during the first pregnancy go on to have healthy subsequent pregnancies. Having heard this, I felt much better. I opted not to have a D & C.

After receiving a prescription for pain medication and literature on the subject of Early Pregnancy Loss, I was advised to wait approximately three months before conceiving again. Jerome met me in the lobby and was rendered speechless by the news. He never would have guessed that an impending miscarriage was what sent me to the doctor's office in such a haste. He accompanied me home and assured me that our next pregnancy would be a success. I wish he had consulted God before making this declaration. I wish we both had.

CHAPTER FOUR

Take Two

What I had experienced was likely a chemical pregnancy. Chemical pregnancies occur shortly after implantation and often result in bleeding that occurs at the time a woman expects a menstrual period. Chemical pregnancies account for more than 50% of miscarriages.

After I recovered physically from the miscarriage, it was back to business as usual. I returned to my normal routine and awaited my next positive pregnancy test. One thing that holds true is that spiritual growth comes at a price. While I was sitting idle and waiting for this perfect plan to manifest, I should have been getting into God's word and asking Him to reveal His plan. I leaned on my own understanding, and according to *my* understanding, this plan should have played out the way Jerome and I intended for it to. I didn't realize that I was at the onset of a serious test of faith. Just as we are tested to earn credentials, we must be tested, broken even, before we can truly affirm our faith in God. How and when those tests come is all a part of God's plan, a plan we cannot alter. God needs to know that when it is all said and done, we will lean on Him.

It wasn't until May of 2003 that my next pregnancy was confirmed. The fact that the pregnancy was confirmed was a feat within itself. After all, my first confirmed pregnancy had ended in miscarriage before I even knew I had conceived.

This was an exciting time, to say the least. Shortly before learning of the pregnancy, Jerome and I had moved in with my mother so we could begin house hunting. During this time I was asked to be a bridesmaid in the wedding of one of my sorority sisters who was to be wed on June 28, 2003.

Notwithstanding my constant bouts with nausea, I was extremely excited about my newly confirmed pregnancy. Just the mere thought of being a mother by January propelled me into a state of euphoria. What an awesome time! We were looking for a house. I was making plans to be in my friend's wedding. Mostly, I was enjoying the time I spent with my little brother and nephew, who were ages 5 and 3, respectively. I could not wait to introduce them to their new little playmate. What could possibly go wrong? I was quickly approaching my second trimester, and the pregnancy was going quite well.

My daily episodes of morning sickness could not obliterate my intense joy. I could not help thinking how awesome God was. It is rather interesting how we are so quick to point out how good God is when all seems well. The truth of the matter is that God is *always* good, and His mercy does indeed endure forever. It seems that we often take His goodness for granted when we are not in the midst of storms. Sometimes God has to get our attention. Sometimes we have to do a little suffering in the process. Sometimes the storms will rage against us, and the storms will subside. However, they will subside in God's way and in His time.

Although my pregnancy was progressing well, Dr. Robinson was keeping close watch on a uterine fibroid that was about the size of a lemon. It had been discovered during one of my ultrasounds. His primary concern was that fibroids tend to increase in size during pregnancy because of the hormone levels. This fibroid had not grown much and had not presented any major problems for me.

Seeking to better understand what was going on with my body, I did my own research on uterine fibroids and found that they are classified according to where they are positioned. They can grow within the wall of the uterus, in the uterine cavity, or outside the uterine wall. Some fibroids, known as pedunculated fibroids, are attached to the uterus by stalk-like growths. The size and location of a fibroid can even impact a woman's ability to conceive. This fibroid, which was growing in the wall of my uterus, had not prevented me from conceiving, but it was still something we needed to watch closely.

When thinking of memorable events, those occurrences leaving indelible marks on our minds and in our hearts, we can almost always remember the defining moment when we knew something was afoot. This situation was no different. It was the morning of June 26, 2003. It was a Thursday morning. I can recall this because Jerome and I were scheduled to travel to Augusta, GA the following day for my sorority sister, Kaci's, wedding.

I was going about my usual morning routine. We were residing with my mother, and her home was full of life in the mornings. There was my 3-year-old nephew and my 5-year-old brother with their laundry list of questions, their adorable laughter, and that zest for life that was characteristic of happy, healthy children.

I had already gotten dressed for work but had to use the restroom. I immediately noticed that I was bleeding. It was not the copious flow I had seen on that unforgettable day in October 2002, but it was alarming just the same. After all, it was never good to see blood flow during pregnancy. I had this sinking feeling in my stomach as I walked into Yashica's room to tell her what was going on. I phoned Jerome, who had already left for work and asked him to return home. As I waited for him to return home, I began to cry. I knew something was wrong. I didn't speak the words into the atmosphere, but I just knew something was wrong.

Once Jerome arrived, I told Yashica that she could go on to work. Jerome and I waited for the doctor's office to open before calling. I just did not feel up to dealing with an answering service. As I lay across the bed, I thought of the miscarriage I had experienced several months before. I also thought about my walk with God. I needed to be close to Him, and I was beginning to wonder if I truly knew how to achieve that closeness. I desperately needed His assurance that this pregnancy would be okay. Jerome sat beside me, rubbing my back. Before we called the doctor's office, Jerome took me by the hand and prayed for our unborn baby.

It came as no surprise that we were advised to report to the doctor's office immediately. After thoroughly examining me and administering an ultrasound, Dr. Robinson assured me that everything appeared to be okay. He warned, however, that I should stay off my feet for the next few days. When I informed him of my plans to participate in a wedding in Augusta, he strongly advised against taking the trip. Against his advice, I honored my commitment to serve as a bridesmaid in the wedding.

Upon my return from the wedding, I felt fine and experienced no more bleeding. While I was still experiencing morning sickness, it had gotten some better. I gave much time and thought to God's goodness. He was showing favor in my life, and I had so much to be grateful for. As I reflected on the miscarriage I had had and the scare I experienced just before Kaci's wedding, I realized that God was strengthening my faith walk and perfecting me to fulfill a greater purpose than I could ever imagine. What I didn't realize was just how much my faith would be tested and how much *strengthening* my faith walk really needed.

Jerome and I had set aside Sunday afternoons for spending quality time together and for house hunting. I came to look forward to this time with my husband as it provided a unique opportunity for us to talk and just bond. We even shared a few laughs along the way. I don't believe he realized how comforting his outer strength was to me. No matter what had come our way, he was courageous and optimistic.

On this particular Sunday afternoon, the sun shone brightly. By all accounts, it was a beautiful July day. The jovial sound of children playing filled the air. Jerome and I set about our usual routine. We hopped into the car and traveled to Richmond Hill, Port Wentworth, and South Effingham County. As we identified homes we wished to inquire about, I was tasked with recording contact numbers.

Still experiencing the occasional stint with morning sickness, I was feeling a little nauseated on this particular day. I even brought along a towel and pillow. Because I so looked forward to our Sunday outings, I made a concerted effort to mask the unusual feeling that suddenly scourged my body.

The nausea was not as bothersome anymore because I had accepted it as a normal occurrence during pregnancy. It was the other feeling that greatly concerned me. There was a dull, constant pain in my lower abdomen, a pain that could easily be compared to a mild menstrual cramp. While the pain was not severe, it did contribute to the discomfort I felt throughout our ride. Even repositioning myself on the pillow failed to provide any substantial relief.

Jerome, keenly aware that I was not feeling well, consistently asked if I was okay and even offered to cut our outing short so that I could go home and rest. I insisted on pressing forward. Prior to returning home, we stumbled over Park West, a new subdivision in South Guyton. There were only a few ranch-style homes, most of which were models. There was something endearing about this quiet subdivision tucked away just west of Savannah. We decided to record the contact information and plan to schedule an appointment to view some of the properties.

The pain in my lower abdomen went from dull to moderate. Having no relief by Monday, I decided to take a day of sick leave. By Monday evening, I had contacted Dr. Robinson and requested something for the pain.

Our appointment with Park West Homes had been scheduled for Tuesday evening at 6:00pm. I decided it would be best for me to spend one more day at home. This would give me ample opportunity to rest, take something for the pain, make our appointment, and be ready to return to work on Wednesday morning. Sounded like a perfect plan of attack, right? Wrong! As God's perfect will would have it, something was definitely afoot. As we walked through the various models and discussed the homes, I was one step from a limp.

I was excited because we decided to pursue a contract on a newly constructed home in the Park West subdivision. The excitement was clouded, however, by this pain that had plagued me for the past several days. It was the type of menacing pain that would take one's breath away. I had made every effort to maintain some sense of normalcy, and I did not want anyone, especially Jerome, to know the full extent of the pain I was feeling.

I had decided that come what may, I would report to work on Wednesday morning. As morning arrived, I held to my decision. Still feeling badly, I moved around rather slowly. Jerome left for work a little early because he had meetings scheduled in Jesup, GA. My mother had traveled to Swainsboro, GA to spend a few days with my grandmother. With everyone gone, the house was quiet, and the morning was uneventful.

Upon arriving at work, I realized that the pain was intense enough to inhibit my ability to function. There was significant cramping, but there was something else, something extremely peculiar. I had a feeling of heaviness in my lower abdomen. It was as if my abdominal area had been stuffed with water balloons. I moved about slowly as if I expected one of the balloons to fall out. I sat at my desk and began to pray quietly. It was at this very location, just nine months prior, that I began to miscarry my first pregnancy. It was like déjà vu.

No longer able to hide the pain, I began to cry. One co-worker invited me into her office to pull myself together. She even alerted my supervisor that I was in great pain and probably needed to go home. As much as I hated to miss a third day from work, I absolutely could not function. I decided to return home.

Once I arrived home, I decided to take a nap. Unfortunately, the pain was not letting up. I paced the floor and even soaked in a tub of warm water. It was simply amazing how still and peaceful the house seemed while this storm was raging inside of me.

I prayed, and I prayed. Then I prayed some more, asking God to do as His word said and give me the desires of my heart. I had never been so afraid or felt so alone in my life. There I was, 14 weeks pregnant feeling like I was in labor. I was so afraid, primarily because I was at home alone. It is an awful feeling realizing you have no control over what is happening to you.

No matter what I did, I found no relief. I sat. I walked. I placed a warm cloth against my abdomen. I prayed. I cried. I asked why this was happening to me. I even questioned where God was during this painful ordeal.

In the midst of my raging storm, I was struck by the most indescribable pain ever. The pain I had felt back in October paled in comparison. On the heels of this excruciating pain was my sudden urge to push. By this time, I had knelt on all fours and was crying out.

"Lord, help me! Please, God, help me!"

The urge to push grew more intense. Having no other recourse, I pulled myself from the floor and sat on the toilet. I was on the toilet for less than 10 seconds when my body began to push, almost involuntarily. I pushed, and I screamed. Then, there it was. There was a feeling of something "popping." The pop was followed by an abundant flow of blood.

I literally crawled to the kitchen to get the phone. I called Dr. Robinson's office to let them know I was on my way. It was by the grace of God that I was able to drive myself there. In my condition, I really should have been transported by ambulance. I can't think of another time that I was so afraid to be behind the wheel. Upon arriving at the doctor's office, I was told that Dr. Robinson was on vacation and that I would be seeing his partner. At that point, I didn't care which doctor I saw, just so I saw one quickly.

Accompanied by a nurse, Dr. Robinson's partner entered the examination room and very cordially introduced himself to me. I managed to crack a small smile as I acknowledged him. Given the emergency nature of my situation, he wasted no time beginning his examination. It took less than a minute for him to conclude that I was experiencing a miscarriage. Although this fact had become apparent to me, hearing the words aloud gave life to it.

"Mrs. Stanton, I am going to attempt to remove as much tissue as possible, but I want to send you for a D & C."

I said absolutely nothing. I just lay on the examination table, crying. The nurse, nearly in tears herself, asked if she could call someone for me. Remembering that my mother and husband were both out of town, I asked her to call my sister.

After a few moments, the doctor looked at me and informed me that I had delivered the baby. He went on to ask me if I wanted to see it. Did I want to see *it*? What was supposed to be my son or daughter had been reduced to a lifeless fetus, passed in an examination room in an OB/GYN office. Wow! I declined the opportunity at a glimpse of my tiny fetus, a decision I sometimes question, even now. What did a fetus look like at 14 weeks' gestation? Could the gender be determined? In a split second, I made a decision that would forever preclude me from knowing the answers to these questions.

Yashica, having been contacted by the nurse, rushed over from work and drove me to Candler Hospital to undergo a D & C. As I was being processed, she contacted Jerome, my mother, and my closest friends. Jerome quickly made his way from Jesup and arrived just in time to kiss me on the forehead as I was being wheeled into the operating room.

A D & C, short for dilation and curettage, can serve multiple purposes. In addition to being used to diagnose or treat such problems as abnormal uterine bleeding, it is used to ensure that all tissue has been completely expelled from the uterus following miscarriages and induced abortions. I had opted not to undergo the procedure following my first miscarriage, but by this pregnancy being further along, it was thought best.

I don't remember much after Jerome's forehead kiss, but what I do recall is awakening in the recovery room and immediately being assured that the procedure had gone well. I would be able to go home that afternoon. That almost seemed like an oxymoron. To say that the procedure had gone well was to say that my pregnancy was officially over…at just 14 weeks! It's almost like saying that all crime-prevention programs had been an amazing success, and there was almost no crime to report. While this would be great news to the affected community, it would stifle the job security of law enforcement professionals. So, having a successful D & C was great from a medical standpoint, but it gave a certain finality to this, my second pregnancy loss.

As Jerome was driving me home, Yashica phoned to inform me that two of my sorority sisters, who were also close friends, were flying down from Atlanta to be with me. I was surprised and extremely touched by this gesture. One notion that holds true is that it's easy for people to be your friends and to gravitate towards you when you're at your best, but you find the true worth in your friendships when you're at your worst.

As I sat on my mother's sofa, chatting with Lisa and Lorrie, I had a myriad of random thoughts. I thought of how selfless it was for these two ladies to drop everything in the middle of the week to come and be with me. I thought about how blessed I was to be surrounded by people who genuinely cared about me. I thought about myself, wondering if I had always been the kind of friend I now so desperately needed. I thought about the unmerited favor God was demonstrating in my life.

It was only a matter of time, though, before my thoughts shifted to the very event that had brought us together on this Wednesday evening. I had just suffered my second miscarriage. I had lost my precious baby – again. So, the God that blessed me with a discerning spirit regarding friendship was the same God I was questioning, but depending on so desperately. I needed Him to help me understand what was happening to me and why *me*. As my mind raced, I thought of a passage of scripture that described what I was feeling:

My God, my God, why hast thou forsaken me? why art thou so far from helping me, and from the words of my roaring? (Psalm 22:1)

I had no answers and very little hope. I even tortured myself by searching for reasons. While I was happy to be surrounded by family and friends, I was consumed with melancholy thoughts. Prior to heading back to Atlanta the following morning, Lisa looked me square in the eye and asked me what I was feeling. She asked if I was hurt or angry. I did not know how to tell her that I could not describe my feelings in a way that she could ever understand. I could never make her understand my deflated faith. Somehow, I felt I had to protect those closest to me from my dejected state of mind. I had to appear to be strong so they would not worry about me. With a face of stone, I responded to my friend.

"I'm going to be okay."

Faith Tested. Truth Revealed. Destiny Fulfilled.

Maybe if I said it loud enough, my heart would believe it to be true. Maybe. Someday. Somehow. Just maybe.

CHAPTER FIVE

Under the Knife... Over the Hurdle

In 2002, Jerome and I had set the perfect plan in motion, and there we were two years later, wondering what had gone wrong. We were left with questions. We were left with overwhelming feelings of grief and loss. We were left with a faltering faith. The only thing we didn't have to show for the tumultuous journey we had taken was a healthy baby. Sure we had been pregnant three times, but there was no pitter patter of little feet. There was no laughter, no cute little facial expressions. There was no baby. I began to wonder if this was my fate. As much as I adored children, maybe motherhood was not in the cards for me.

As I pondered my maternal fate, I began to reflect on the events that had occurred over the past two years. Only a fraction of my thoughts were of the precious babies I had lost. I also thought of my friends and family. I couldn't help thinking of the beautiful, healthy babies who had been born to close friends while I was in the fight of my life.

I can specifically recall a beautiful, sunny day in September 2003. It had been less than two months since my second miscarriage. I was driving along Abercorn Street when my cell phone rang.

"Hello, Stacy? This is Keith."

Keith is the husband of one of my closest friends, Kisha. When I heard his voice, I immediately knew why he was calling. He was calling to tell me that their second son, Keith, Jr., had been born.

"Do we have a baby?" I asked excitedly.

"Yes, we have a baby!"

Keith sounded excited, and there was no reason he should not have been. He had a new, perfectly healthy baby boy. He went on to tell me the baby's length and weight and that Kisha and the baby were doing great. I told Keith that I would give Kisha time to rest and would call her a little later. Kisha had officially completed her family, and I could not have been happier for her. She was a beautiful person who was so deserving of this blessing.

All I wanted was for my friends to have healthy, successful pregnancies. I wanted them to realize their dreams of motherhood. As much as I wanted this for them, I wanted it for myself. In God's infinite wisdom, He was not allowing my dream to manifest. As I reflected, I thought of all the possible reasons my body could be failing me. What was it about my body that was preventing me from doing the one thing every woman should be able to do? What I had not considered at this juncture was the possibility that it had nothing to do with my body and everything to do with God's divine plan.

When Jerome arrived home, I shared the good news with him.

"Kisha had the baby today!"

"She did? That's great!"

It is crazy. Within moments of sharing this awesome news with Jerome, I was in tears. This was a time of rejoicing, and there I was, crying uncontrollably. Jerome wrapped his arms around me.

"Baby, I know what's bothering you. It's going to be okay. Our day is coming."

All I could do was nod. I was amazed at how I never had to tell him when I needed to be encouraged. I lay there, thinking of Kisha's baby. I lay there, thinking of Lisa's baby, who was due to arrive in April 2004. I lay there, thinking of my friend Kim's baby, who was due to arrive in February 2004. I prayed that God would not leave me alone in this desolate place that is infertility. I prayed that He would allow me to know the joy people all around me were feeling – the joy of motherhood.

*   *   *

A couple of weeks after Angel's demise, I was preparing for a follow-up doctor's appointment. My home was quiet as Jerome had returned to work. I was left alone with my thoughts, so I did what any grieving mother would do. I reached for something that would bring me closer to Angel. I went to my closet and pulled out the little box I had been given at the hospital. For the rest of my life, this box would be the only proof I had that Angel ever existed, and I would hold on to it with everything in me.

I untied the dark green ribbon slowly and opened the box. The first item I pulled out was a little white dress that had been hand sewn by the Waving Girls Chapter of the Smocking Arts Guild of America. On the lower left corner of the dress was the cutest little embroidered pink dog. This adorable dress had been placed on my precious baby after her death so she could be photographed. The hospital staff even placed a pink hat on her head to match the dog on the dress. It was also in the box. A picture of Angel wearing this dress and hat was accompanied by a picture that had been taken immediately after her birth. In this picture, Angel was wearing the standard pink and blue hat that is placed on all newborns. She was also wearing a hospital bracelet bearing my name, the doctor's name, and her birth date and time. Her head was tilted slightly to the left, and her tiny left hand was nestled just under her left cheek.

These pictures managed to tug at my aching heart each time I fixed my eyes on them. The memory box was filled with heartfelt sympathy and get-well cards and a book titled *When a Baby Dies*. Further investigation of the box yielded two documents from Fox & Weeks Funeral Home, the funeral home that had handled Angel's cremation. One document was an authorization for cremation and the other, the certificate of cremation. By the time I read Angel's confirmation of birth and made my way to the bottom of the box where I kept her ultrasound pictures, I was blinded by tears. How could this be happening? Was God punishing me? Was He trying to get my attention? If so, why? Why were my friends having these healthy, full-term babies while I was battling infertility with all I had? I wasn't sad because they were having successful pregnancies. I was sad because I wasn't.

As I tied the green, satin ribbon, I sat holding my little box of Angel's memories. At that moment, it occurred to me that something needed to change. The old adage tells us that if we keep doing what we're doing, we'll keep getting the same result. Something definitely had to change. I knew I needed to change my approach from a medical perspective, but I didn't realize that I needed a change from a *spiritual* perspective as well. I needed to hear from God, but at the height of my grief, I just didn't know how to go to Him. I thought I did, but I was quickly learning that there was a significant piece missing from the puzzle.

The joy and excitement I once felt during prenatal visits had given way to feelings of awkwardness, anxiety and shame. The waiting room was always full of young, vibrant, pregnant ladies. There I was, the 31-year-old woman who could not even carry a pregnancy to term. Although these young ladies knew nothing of my situation, I was terribly embarrassed.

"We probably need to consider getting that thing out of there," Dr. Robinson said as I sat on the examination table.

I had learned from him that my lemon-sized uterine fibroid had grown to be nearly twice the size of my uterus. He explained to me that while he was delivering Angel, he removed a small, pedunculated fibroid. Removing the larger one would not be that simple. He went on to explain that trying to remove a fibroid that large while in the middle of another major surgery could result in a greater loss of blood and increase the risk of a hysterectomy.

"The procedure to remove the larger fibroid is called a myomectomy," he continued, "and it could possibly increase your chance of carrying a pregnancy full term."

"How soon can we do this?" I wanted to get this out of the way as soon as possible and get back to the business at hand, becoming a mother.

Dr. Robinson, in his professional and thorough manner, insisted that I understand that having this surgery in no way guaranteed a positive outcome. While removing the fibroid seemed to be the most logical course of action, the procedure was not without serious risks. Dr. Robinson encouraged me to actively participate in my care by educating myself on the risk factors involved in undergoing a myomectomy.

My case was particularly delicate because the goal was to keep the uterus completely intact. After all, the key purpose behind everything we did was to ensure my ability to have children. To that end, maintaining the health of my uterus was critical. Some of the risks involved included excessive blood loss, development of scar tissue, and complications in subsequent pregnancies. Whew! Was this something I really wanted to do? Had I not experienced enough pregnancy complications and blood loss? I had a major decision to make, and it was not going to be an easy one.

Out of desperation, I had given a rather hasty response to Dr. Robinson when he advised that I consider a myomectomy. I'm thankful that he halted me and encouraged me to give careful thought to the benefits and drawbacks of having this major abdominal surgery. This was definitely not a time to make hasty, impolitic decisions.

I prayed for guidance. I prayed that God would show favor, regardless of what I decided. It would be a gross understatement to say that I was afraid. I had come against a force much larger than myself, and I think I was finally starting to understand the importance of going to God earnestly and sincerely and just seeking His face. I was afraid to have the surgery. I was afraid *not* to have the surgery. I was gripped with fear and uncertainty. If I had the surgery, I could risk permanent infertility. If I *didn't* have the surgery, I could risk permanent infertility. I was at a place where I didn't know where to turn or what to do. As strange as it may seem, that is just where God needed me. He needed me in a place where I could rely totally on Him and hear His voice. God could not manifest His purpose in my life if I did not totally submit to His will. As I pondered my decision, I was comforted by the following passage of scripture:

For God hath not given us a spirit of fear; but of power, and of love, and of a sound mind. (2 Timothy 1:7)

It was that power and that sound mind that ultimately led me to a decision. After researching the risks, discussing it with Jerome, and most importantly, seeking God, I decided to proceed with the surgery. Dr. Robinson assured me that extra care would be taken to ensure my uterus remained intact. He would even be accompanied by a reproductive endocrinologist with extensive experience performing myomectomies. To allow adequate time to fully recover from my cesarean delivery, we decided to have the surgery in July, just four months after my unpalatable experience with Angel.

Dr. Robinson conveyed to me the importance of not becoming pregnant prior to the surgery. He obviously could not perform the surgery if I were pregnant. Although I fully understood the gravity of this matter, I could not help feeling like I was moving backwards. There I was, trying so hard to become a mother. Now, I had to suspend my efforts until after this surgery that might or might not make a difference. The four months I spent awaiting my surgery seemed like four years. On several occasions, I seriously considered canceling the surgery and just accepting what seemed like the inevitable. I wanted to wait on God, but I also wanted to do all I could.

During the time that I was waiting to have surgery, my childhood best friend moved back to Savannah. Stephanie had just completed graduate school at the University of Georgia and desired to live closer to her mother. I was ecstatic that she was returning to the Savannah area, and her return could not have come at a better time.

Stephanie and I have a friendship that dates back to 1985 when we were energetic, know-it-all preteens. We have seen the best and worst of times in our lives together, and I have often drawn on her seemingly unfaltering strength to cope with life's challenges. Even someone with Stephanie's resolve was often at a loss for words when hearing of my struggle with infertility. She told me on several occasions that she felt inadequate because she just didn't know what to say or do to comfort me. What she didn't realize was having her back home helped a great deal. Although I had settled into my decision to undergo surgery, I was still somewhat afraid, so it was great to have Stephanie here to talk to.

My surgery took place on July 21, 2004. The monstrous fibroid, which was almost twice the size of my uterus, was successfully removed. As I rested, I listened carefully to Dr. Robinson's report.

"It was impressive. It was very large. Some parts of it had started to degenerate, which essentially means those cells were dying and could have released chemicals that could have caused severe pain."

"So, what is my prognosis?"

Dr. Robinson indicated that he could not have been more pleased with the procedure. The fibroid was gone. My uterus was completely intact, and there should be very little scar tissue. The prognosis was positive. Motherhood just might be in the cards for me after all. God hadn't forgotten about me. I was just getting my second wind. I had a minor setback, but with the removal of that fibroid came the restoration of my waning faith in miracles. This was my time, or was it?

CHAPTER SIX

Walking Out of the Valley

As I recovered from my myomectomy, I was increasingly optimistic about my prognosis. I began to thank God for the storm I had just experienced. This storm unleashed a sense of strength and determination that had been dormant in my spirit. I almost gave up on my dream of having a child of my own and giving Jerome the child he so desired, but this experience landed me in a good place, a place of promise. My faith, which was extremely unsound just a few months prior, had been revitalized as a withering flower invigorated by the touch of nature's rain. My body was healthy. My faith had been restored, and I was back in the game.

Amidst my immoderate optimism, something very unsettling happened. Seemingly without warning, I slipped into a state of utter depression. I cannot say with unmitigated certainty that I was clinically depressed, but I definitely showed some clear signs. I was no longer jovial at the thought of motherhood. My emotions alternated between fear, embarrassment, sadness, and loneliness. I knew this was not a healthy array of feelings, but I found a way to rationalize them.

I had spent so much time masking my feelings in a flimsy attempt at appearing okay. I never wanted those close to me to see me crying, so I suppressed the tears until I was alone. I didn't want anyone feeling sorry for me or protective over me. I didn't want to be treated as though my heart needed to be guarded. I just wanted to be a normal young woman with goals to achieve and dreams to fulfill. I didn't want to appear different. I didn't want to stand out. I kept at the task of building a wall around my heart. When looking at me, people saw strength. They saw a steadfast, spiritually and emotionally grounded woman who was in complete control of her destiny. I definitely didn't look like what I had been through.

The truth of the matter was that I viewed myself as a beautiful spirit housed in a defective shell. My body, my temple, was unable to do the very thing a woman boasts of being able to do – perpetuate human life. I carried a heavy burden. I carried grief for the babies I had lost. I carried the shame of not being able to bring forth new life. I carried the daunting fear that I might never be able to carry a pregnancy to full term. On occasion, I even carried envy for my friends, for my sister, and for the women all over the world who were doing what comes naturally for a woman. Why could I not do this? I had never carried the green-eyed monster on my back before. These burdensome feelings definitely represented uncharted territory for me.

If a girlfriend told me she had purchased a new car, I congratulated her. A new house? Wonderful! Academic achievement? You go girl! I could cheer her on like it was my news, but it was something about hearing her say, "I'm pregnant!" that made me cringe.

For so long, I had hidden from the world how inadequate I felt. What would my friends think of me if they knew there were days I didn't want to hear about that cute comment little Johnny had made? How would they feel if they knew how many times I had gotten off the phone with them and cried a river?

I walked around pretending to be a pillar of strength. I kept telling myself that God does not make mistakes, but unless I believed that statement, it was just a useless cliché. I can recall the morning after I lost Angel. My pastor visited me in the hospital, and during his stay, he recited for me, Romans 8:28, the very same scripture that appeared at the beginning of the book I had received from Ms. Louise the day before. He went on to ask me if I was angry with God. I found the question rather unsettling. What kind of maniacal person actually admitted to being angry with God? I guess I believed not saying it out loud made it less true. I'm not sure if what I was feeling was anger, but it was definitely a spiritual disengagement of sorts.

For nearly two years, I had put my best on the outside and done a pretty impressive job of hiding my true feelings. Now, every emotion surrounding my struggle with infertility was disgorged from my body like a piece of food being expelled by way of the Heimlich Maneuver. Was I angry with God? I don't know, but I couldn't help wondering how He could allow me to suffer two miscarriages only to have my newborn baby die just hours after birth? Hadn't I said the right prayers? Hadn't I believed? The Bible tells us that faith comes by hearing, and I was in the sanctuary as often as possible to hear what thus said the Lord. If it wasn't His plan for me to be a mother, why had He allowed me to become pregnant over and over? I was confused. I was hurt, and I was tired of pretending to be okay.

I wanted to scream to anyone within the sound of my voice, "I'm not okay! I want my babies! I just wish I had my babies!"

Even the excitement I exuded after my myomectomy was a cover. While I was grateful that the surgery had gone well, I was sadly overwhelmed by the events that preceded the surgery. I could no longer hide my emotions. I began to wear them on my sleeve, and I stopped caring who knew.

I spent many hours in deep thought, often wondering what other people thought of my situation. Was I viewed as a basket case? Were people feeling sorry for me? I had become a statistic. I wore a label. Should that label have been stamped on my forehead? I sometimes felt it had been.

"I am infertile," I should have announced when meeting new people. Maybe that would have helped us avoid the awkwardness that arose when asked why Jerome and I had not started a family.

I thought of Jerome often, wondering if he realized the depth of my pain. I mean, it was my body that had felt the babies move. It was me who had failed miserably at carrying a pregnancy to full term. Although we discussed the specific events, we both avoided speaking in great detail about our feelings. Although Jerome never outwardly made me feel that any of this was my fault, I sometimes wondered if he felt that way. On the morning after Angel's demise, I was left to dissect my feelings of grief while Jerome took some time to himself. I so desperately wanted to know how he felt. Was he pulling away from me because I could not save Angel, or was he grieving privately so he could be strong when in my presence?

Because lengthy, involved discussions of Angel's death fostered an environment of awkwardness, we often avoided them. To that end, I sometimes felt that our decision to cremate her was too premature. We weren't thinking clearly, and we weren't communicating as we should have been. Neither of us wanted to have an emotional breakdown in the presence of the other. Unlike the miscarriages, this was not something we could just sweep under the rug and move past. Our little girl had died. She was real, and the feelings of grief and loss surrounding her transition were extremely real. How do two people so stricken with grief help each other along the path of healing? They don't. They enlist God's help.

I prayed for myself. I prayed for a clearer understanding of the process Jerome was going through. There he was, my husband, my protector, feeling inadequate. He felt this way because he wanted to be there for me but had his own cross to bear.

I can remember being on the table in the operating room and hearing the faint voices that encompassed me. What I wanted to know, though, was what that picture looked like from Jerome's perspective. After all, he wasn't incoherent like I was. He wasn't sedated. He was fully alert which likely placed him at a disadvantage. For him, the picture was clear, vivid, colorful, and unimaginably tragic. He told me he remembered the moment Angel arrived, struggling to take her first breath. He remembered Dr. Robinson hurriedly handing her over to the staff of the Neonatal Intensive Care Unit (NICU). She was tiny, fragile, beautiful, sick, peaceful – so many things at once.

Jerome spoke of the moment she was placed in his arms. She was soft and warm, and her heart was racing. He so desperately wanted to breathe life into her. He wondered how he was supposed to let his little girl go and help his wife do the same. What an enormous burden to bear!

As we traveled along our emotional roller coaster, the days turned into weeks and the weeks into months. I was back to some semblance of normalcy, but I thought of my babies often, especially Angel. I thought of how I almost died giving birth to her and still wasn't able to save her. I thought of the surgery. I thought of everything all the time. While thinking, I began to write. In the process, I penned this poem as a tribute to my babies:

The Ones

The ones we never cried for
In our haste to fill the void
Our little miscarried and unborn angels
We sent back up to the Lord

The ones we gave no names to
Or held close to our bosoms with glee
The ones whose spirits left us
Before their faces we could see

The ones who cry out in darkness
To let us know that they are there
The ones who remind us daily
That God only gives what we can bear

The ones who never grabbed Mommy's hand
So she could ease their fears
The ones who never scraped their knees
And let Mommy dry their tears

The ones who never had a piggy back ride
Mounted safely on Daddy's back
The ones he never bounced in the air
Or walked to school with little backpacks

The ones we never taught to spell
Or to count from one to ten
The ones we never taught sportsmanship
And how to graciously lose or win

The ones who were plucked from the garden
Before their seeds could fully mature
The ones who strengthened our faith
And taught Mommy and Daddy to endure

The ones we would have been so proud of
With their faces like Daddy and me
The ones who left us crying
Lord, why'd my babies leave me?

Their little bodies didn't last long
But their spirits will live always
The ones I will carry in my heart
Throughout all my days

I will share my strength with other mommies
Whose babies' feet never touched the ground
Our little miscarried and unborn angels
Whose little voices never made a sound.

I realized I needed some way to channel this abundance of emotion. I needed an outlet. I was wearing grief like a cloak. Every time I saw a baby, I slipped into that melancholy place. I would look at other women and wonder what made them different. Wasn't I just as healthy, just as deserving? I just did not understand God's message in all this. What I did understand, however, was that I needed some way to escape the pain. I had this overwhelming need to feel I was doing something that mattered.

One day, as I sat alone with my thoughts, I had an epiphany. I thought about something Yashica had done about a month after Angel's death. She called and proclaimed that she had a gift for me. The glee in her voice told me she was sure this gift would cheer me up.

"I'm going to send you a link to a website, and I want you to call me once you've seen it."

"What is it?" I asked, still not completely excited.

"Just check your e-mail and call me back."

"Okay."

Without hesitation, I checked my e-mail account and clicked on the link my sister had referred to. As the page loaded, I noticed a picture of her. Upon further perusal, I realized the page was for the annual fundraising event for the March of Dimes. Yashica had signed up as an individual participant to honor Angel's memory. I stared at the webpage, repeatedly reading Yashica's blurb about Angel and why Angel's story had inspired her to participate in WalkAmerica. The tears began to fall. I cried because of this selfless thing my sister had done. I also cried because I realized that there were millions of "Angels" out there.

The March of Dimes is really a remarkable organization, whose funding and research successfully alleviated polio before they turned their attention to the prevention of prematurity, birth defects, and infant mortality. Their largest annual fundraiser, WalkAmerica, recently became known as the March for Babies. Maybe their hard work couldn't save Angel, but one day I wouldn't feel her death was in vain.

Within two weeks, Yashica managed to raise more than $500 in the fight for the healthy delivery of all babies. On April 24, 2004, she and Jerome joined thousands of walkers from the Savannah area for a 6-mile walk. I could not have been more proud!

As I sat and thought of ways to cope, I realized that this was a great way to channel my feelings of loss. I would continue what Yashica had started. I decided to form a team to honor Angel's memory. Maybe one day, like polio, we would get a handle on premature births and infant mortality. We affectionately called our team the Earth Angels and began to recruit family and friends to participate. Being a team captain for an event like this can be mentally taxing, but the thought of helping other affected families while honoring my daughter's memory was just the fuel I needed to press on.

On April 30, 2005, the Earth Angels Family Team made its debut in the Coastal Empire WalkAmerica event. Our team boasted about 20 walkers and raised approximately $1,500 to help save babies. We donned canary yellow t-shirts with blue lettering. I was even able to pull myself together enough to have Angel's actual footprints printed on the shirts. It was a great day and a great cause. I had already started thinking of the 2006 event.

Having learned more about the March of Dimes programs, my ambition intensified for the 2006 event. This was evident by the significant increase in participants. On April 29, 2006, with more than 40 participants, the Earth Angels had a strong presence. I had even appeared on a local news program, Coastal Sunrise, with the Executive Director of the local March of Dimes chapter. The event was a Herculean success for our team, who raised more than $6,000. Of all teams participating, including local hospitals and many corporate teams, we placed fifth. I had the honor of meeting mothers who had recently lost their babies or whose babies were still in the NICU. Being able to encourage these women was absolutely priceless.

Shortly after the 2006 event, I was invited to join the NICU Family Support Committee, which provides support for NICU families through activities for siblings, educational seminars, post-NICU follow-up, etc. Becoming involved with the March of Dimes allowed me to take small, but significant steps to *walking* out of the valley.

CHAPTER SEVEN

Evidence of Things Not Seen

Becoming involved with the March of Dimes walk had proven to be extremely therapeutic for me. Although it was an incessant reminder of the trials I had endured, it was rewarding to be able to give back in such a positive way. I needed that, and I was happy that I had decided to do it. It was easy to become consumed with anything that would play an integral role in putting painful thoughts to rest.

Being a woman who could not bear the fruit of life, I could have quite easily maintained a rather dismal existence. I wanted more for myself, and I knew God expected more of me. I had to remember that although my journey to motherhood had taken a few unexpected turns, I was still blessed. I had a wonderfully supportive husband. Notwithstanding my plight with infertility, I was healthy and strong. I had a close-knit, supportive family. I realized that while my faith walk was a constant work in progress, I still had so much to be thankful for. Grumbling, complaining, and throwing myself the occasional proverbial pity party was not going to bring me any closer to my destiny.

As I attended Sunday worship services and Wednesday bible study, I was constantly reminded by my pastor that God often allowed trials as part of the process of building us up to fulfill His purpose in our lives. I had been raised in a Christian home, the granddaughter of a Baptist minister. I had been inundated with scripture throughout my life and could recite the words to just about any hymn. This experience was another glaring reminder that none of those things made me a Christian. None of those things helped build my relationship with God. Having a close, personal relationship with God has nothing to do with how many hymns you know, how many scriptures you can recite, or what type of show you put on during worship service. A relationship with God requires complete submission. It requires the ability to maintain a strong prayer life. It further requires the ability to seek peace when storms rage in our lives.

This trial was helping me to define my relationship with God. It was helping me understand where I had fallen short within that relationship. It's amazing that I didn't even realize at the time how strong my relationship was becoming. I didn't even realize the spiritual transformation I was going through. What I did know was that there was nothing I could do to change my situation, so I *had* to trust God to do it. During this time, there was a passage of scripture that became a maxim by which I began to live. That passage was Romans 5:1-5, which reads:

1 — Therefore being justified by faith, we have peace with God through our Lord Jesus Christ:
2 — By whom also we have access by faith into this grace wherein we stand, and rejoice in hope of the glory of God
3 — And not only so, but we glory in tribulations also: knowing that tribulation worketh patience:
4 — And patience, experience; and experience, hope:
5 — And hope maketh not ashamed; because the love of God is shed abroad in our hearts by the Holy Ghost which is given unto us.

I read this passage almost daily, especially when I found myself losing ground. I wanted to change my way of thinking. I had been questioning God on so many levels, but I needed to trust Him. I needed to trust that standing on His word as a valiant soldier and pushing past my pain, my trials, my heartaches, my setbacks, and my tears would eventually render me the peace and love of God I so desperately wanted and the strength I so desperately needed. Although I was still in transition, I was beginning to better understand.

This period of transition sometimes rendered the most unexpected emotional jolts. In January 2005, as I was busy preparing for our first March of Dimes walk, I learned that Yashica was pregnant with her second child. She delivered the news to me by phone, and I sat holding the receiver in complete shock. In the days that followed, my emotional state alternated between excitement about the new baby that would be joining our family and sadness because I wasn't the one bringing that new baby into the family. I wanted to scream to my sister. I wanted to scream to my friends. I wanted to scream to the passersby on the street whom I didn't even know. I wanted to tell them to have no more babies until I could have my chance. For once, instead of being Auntie Stacy, I just wanted to be Mommy.

I prayed and prayed. I wanted to send the message to God that I was really trying to cope. I was desperately trying, but because having a baby was such a natural part of life, I could not escape the fact that it was taking place all around me all the time. Every time I resolved to embrace the joys of life and not focus on this problem that had become such a thorn in my side, I was reminded of what I was missing out on. There was no escaping this rueful reality that had become my life. I could not seem to have children, but that didn't stop everyone else from doing so.

"Tribulation worketh patience, and patience, experience and experience, hope."

I recited the passage to myself a million times. I needed to know that something wonderful would come of this ordeal. I needed to have faith in miracles. Sometimes, though, I failed miserably at believing.

I made a conscious decision to engulf myself in everything *else* that was going on in my life. In March 2005, I accepted a position at Savannah Technical College as Coordinator of a program that provided services and resources to single parents, single pregnant women, displaced homemakers, nontraditional students, and any other students with significant barriers to completing their education. Services included educational seminars, a lending library, customized training programs and referrals to community agencies, but it largely consisted of offering a listening ear.

For some, this program represented that one last effort to get on the path to a better life. Ironically, God had placed me there to help these clients, most of whom were young ladies, bridge the gap between where they were and where they wanted to be. I would often hear heart wrenching stories of broken dreams and lost hope. I had to be that voice of reason. I had to provide a compelling argument for not giving up. I think this assignment was an opportunity for me to hear what God had to say regarding my own situation as well. After all, how could I encourage these young ladies when I couldn't trust God to move in my situation?

Considering everything I was faced with, I realized that I needed to suspend my grief and focus on the task at hand. I realized that instead of forcing myself to get over the storm, I should pray for the strength to endure the storm. It was not about not feeling the hurt and devastation, but it was about channeling those feelings into positive energy in order to do what I needed to do.

To that end, I became heavily involved in Yashica's pregnancy, even deciding to host the baby shower. I was enjoying my job and was also enjoying our team's moderate success in WalkAmerica. It was a busy time for me, and I was surrounded by positive energy. Even though there were still days when the burden seemed a bit heavy, I pressed on.

Yashica's baby shower was planned for June 25, 2005, and in my usual fashion, I included all of the frills and fancies. There was plenty of food. There were fun games with great prizes. There were also cute souvenirs. It was my hope that my support would be evident.

I was extremely excited about the impending birth of my nephew, and Yashica looked radiant during her pregnancy. She was all belly, not gaining much weight anywhere else. I remember looking at her and wondering what that felt like. What did it feel like to be only one month away from your due date and still be pregnant? Would I ever know? That remained to be seen.

In the month that followed Yashica's baby shower, we began the task of preparing for my nephew's birth. I found myself faced with a very difficult choice. Yashica had asked me to be in the delivery room. She was scheduled to deliver my nephew by cesarean section. I had been in the room to witness the birth of my older nephew, Jayden, in 2000. However, I was in such a different place then. The experience would take on a very different meaning for me this time around. When Jayden was born, I had not begun what would become the cumbersome task of trying to have a baby. I wanted my second nephew's birth to be a time of joy for me and for my family. I thought it would be rather selfish of me to drag my family into one of my pity parties during this time. I was immensely afraid that being in the delivery room would invoke much of what I felt during and after Angel's birth. The goal was to focus on the blessing we were receiving and not on what I had lost.

I know that Yashica would not have wanted me to feel awkward in any way. She only wanted me in the delivery room so that I could support her during the birth of her son. Cesarean deliveries can sometimes be more frightening than vaginal deliveries because the mother is rendered helpless. She is wide awake during a major surgical procedure with only an epidural to protect her from the pain. The only thing that precludes her from actually seeing the doctor make the incision and pull the baby from her womb is a sheet. She has no control over the process, and all she can do is lay there, praying that all is well on the other side of that sheet. Until the moment she feels the pressure of the baby being pulled from her exposed womb, she does not know how the procedure is going. It can be very unnerving. With that in mind, I totally get why Yashica might have wanted me there. I could only hope that she understood why it was more than I could handle. It had only been 16 months since *my* cesarean delivery.

I believe that because I had done such a remarkable job of masking my feelings for so long, people often forgot how difficult this was for me. With every passing day, I was reminded that I had not been able to do my part in completing the family Jerome and I wanted. Because I sent the message that I was always okay, people treated me that way. No one realized the personal hell I was going through. To an extent, that was good because it meant I was succeeding at suppressing my feelings. I never wanted to be treated differently, so I was okay with internalizing my feelings. Although I couldn't be in the delivery room with Yashica, I was happy that she thought I was strong enough to handle it.

God has a way of working everything out. As fate would have it, the baby's father wanted to be in the delivery room. I assured Yashica that I would be in the waiting room awaiting the news of the birth. Seeing all the families in the waiting room, anxious to hear of their new bundles of joy reminded me of the momentous blessing this was. For every family represented, a new life was beginning. How could I not be happy about that? How could I not want that for myself?

At approximately 11:20a.m., on July 27, 2005, my nephew Justin Tyler was born. He was beautiful. He was perfect. He was living proof of how awesome God is. When I held him, I could not have felt more connected to a baby if he were my own. I was glad he had safely transitioned to his new life outside the womb. I was even more pleased that my sister never had to know firsthand what I had been experiencing.

For the next four days, I stayed at Yashica's apartment, making daily trips to the hospital. My mother had to leave two days after Justin's birth, so I decided to stay until Yashica was home from the hospital and settled in with the new baby. I was busy cleaning, assembling the baby's bassinet, and preparing food that Yashica could just pull from the freezer and place in the microwave. I even found the time to take Jayden and Henri to a movie.

On Sunday, July 31st, I did some last-minute tidying as I awaited Yashica's phone call. Because I had planned to return to Savannah that day, I packed up my things and helped the boys pack theirs. The apartment was cleaned, disinfected, and completely baby-ready.

Throughout the day, I carried this heavy emotional burden. I can usually attribute such feelings to thoughts of my fallen angels. This was different somehow. I knew in my spirit that what I was feeling had nothing to do with my babies. I just knew it. I could not offer a plausible explanation for this heavy, melancholy feeling, but I couldn't seem to shake it. I didn't want to admit it at the time, but what I was feeling was eerily similar to the feeling I had the last time I saw my father alive. It was as if I knew something terrible was on the horizon, but I wanted to put it out of my mind.

Despite this feeling, I was excited about picking Yashica and the baby up from the hospital. I had spoken to Yashica several times throughout the day, and I noticed she seemed very agitated. She could not get any clear answers as to why her discharge was taking so long. Finally, at approximately 3:00p.m., she phoned to say she was being released. With Jayden and Henri in tow, I headed for Northside Hospital to retrieve Yashica and Justin.

Although it had been four days since she gave birth, I noticed that Yashica still seemed to be in a considerable amount of pain. Her doctor had written a prescription for pain medication, which we had filled en route to her apartment. Although I know some pain was to be expected, I was a little concerned about the degree of pain four days after delivery.

Upon arriving at her apartment, I helped Yashica get settled in and showed her the food I had prepared. She was pleasantly surprised to see that Justin's bassinet was assembled. Even with all of this going on, it was so difficult for me to ignore this overwhelming combination of sadness and anxiety I was feeling. I even said a little prayer, asking God to cover Yashica in the apartment and to cover me as I traveled back to Savannah with two small children. My prayer was that God would dispatch angels to protect all of us.

Although I was scheduled to return to work the next day, it was so difficult for me to leave. What I felt went beyond general concern for Yashica and the baby. It was almost as if I felt compelled to stay to protect them from some menacing event that was about to occur. I was happy that Jayden would be returning to Savannah so that Yashica could have some time to get used to having a new baby in the home, but I just wanted the two of them to be okay in that apartment.

Disregarding my angst, I prepared to take the trip back to Savannah. I realized that prolonging my departure was not going to help relieve me of my uneasy feelings, so I resolved to stay in prayer and to believe that God would be with all of us. Upon arriving in Savannah, I phoned Yashica to inform her that we had safely arrived. She, in turn, informed me that she had begun to cry shortly after our departure. She had no idea what had brought on her crying spell. Could she have been sharing my anxiety? Maybe she had the same daunting feeling I had that something just was not right. Not wanting to surmise that we were on the brink of a detrimental event of some sort, I concluded that Yashica must have been suffering from baby blues. Baby blues, however, could not account for *my* anxiety as I had not just given birth. Everyone was safe, so I just attempted to put the feelings aside.

As I returned to work on Monday, the day was rather uneventful. I spent much of my time answering e-mails and returning calls that had been placed while I was away. I just wanted to make it through the day so I could get home and get some much needed rest.

As I tossed and turned in bed that night, I tried to ignore the sound of the alarm. I could not muster up enough energy to hit the snooze button. As I turned towards my nightstand and slowly opened my eyes, I immediately zeroed in on the bright, red digits on the clock. They read, "3:23." At that moment, I jumped up, realizing that what I had heard was clearly not the alarm clock. I rubbed my eyes and glanced over at Jerome, who was sound asleep. At that moment, I heard it again. I realized that what I thought was the alarm clock had actually been my phone ringing.

Afraid to pick up the phone, I began to shake Jerome.

"Jerome, wake up! Someone's calling, and I'm scared!"

"Who is it?" he asked in a groggy voice.

"I don't know! I'm scared to answer!"

I was absolutely petrified. It was as if I knew I was about to learn what my constant anxiety had been about.

I slowly picked up the receiver and pressed the "talk" button. By then, the person had hung up, but a voice mail message had been left. I played the message back.

"Stacy, call me as soon as you get this message!"

The nervous voice I heard was my mother's. Just as my heart was about to jump out of the t-shirt I was wearing, I heard her mumble something as she was hanging up the phone. After replaying the message twice, I was able to decipher what she had said.

"Lord, please help my child," she uttered just as she was hanging up the phone.

"Oh, God," I thought, "What in the world was going on? Was it Henri? Was he having trouble breathing? What was happening?"

I managed to stop shaking long enough to dial my mother's number. She answered on the first ring.

"Hey, Stacy," she said, still sounding very anxious.

"What's wrong?"

"Shica's in that apartment sick. She needs an ambulance. Do you have Toya's number? I'm calling Raymond."

"I'm calling her now!"

I jumped out of the bed and grabbed my cell phone. I was glad my cousin, LaToya's, number was programmed in the phone because I was too nervous to dial. LaToya answered on the first ring.

"Toya, what are you doing?" was all I could say.

"I just talked to Shica. I'm on my way to get her."

"Call 9-1-1 and have the paramedics meet you there!"

"I will call you as soon as I get to her."

I called my mother back, and she told me she had reached my uncle, Raymond, who was also on his way to Yashica's apartment. I was so scared. I began to cry, and then I thought about Justin.

"Oh, God! What about the baby? Where's the baby? What's wrong with my sister?"

I was in my living room by this time, in a fetal position, crying frantically. I didn't have any details. All I knew was that my sister, who was 250 miles away, was very sick and was alone with a 5-day-old baby.

LaToya called back to inform me that she and Uncle Raymond had decided to head to the hospital. They were able to confirm that the paramedics were en route to Yashica's apartment. LaToya said she could hear the distress in my voice and assured me that everything was going to be okay. Although I knew she had no control over whether or not everything would be okay, it was nice to hear the words.

Once we knew LaToya and Raymond were headed to the hospital and that the paramedics were headed to Yashica's, I felt somewhat better. Knowing help was on the way gave me some solace. This was until my mother called back frantically informing me that Yashica had called and said she didn't think she could make it to the door when the paramedics arrived. She was shaking and could not gain enough control to walk, or even crawl, to the door. My first thought was that the fire department could get in the apartment if she couldn't get to the door. With that in mind, I called LaToya back and told her to contact the emergency dispatch and have them send a fire truck out. This was beginning to play out like something in a movie! The only problem was that my sister was no actress and could not just get up and walk off the set should something happen to her.

As the phone calls were exchanged, our family members in Swainsboro were notified of what was going on. In Savannah, we were praying. In Swainsboro, they were praying. In Atlanta, they were praying. We were all praying because we knew my sister needed a move by God to make it safely to the hospital. As my mother prepared to travel to Atlanta, my uncle, Milton, offered to accompany her. Not knowing, or caring, what I would do about childcare, I told my mother to bring Henri and Jayden to me.

LaToya, who had made it to the hospital and was waiting with Uncle Raymond and his wife, Elaine, called me when the paramedics arrived.

"Stacy, they are pulling up now."

"Do you see her?"

"They are wheeling her in. She looks like she is sleeping."

As LaToya was talking to me, Uncle Raymond tried to get as much information from the paramedics as he could while they were rushing Yashica back. What he did learn was that she had been stabilized. I told LaToya to keep me updated as they learned more. She informed me that she was planning to stay right there at the hospital at least until my mother could get to Atlanta.

By the time my mother reached my house with the boys, it was approximately 5:00a.m. She filled me in on her initial call from Yashica. Apparently, she awoke around 2:30a.m. to feed Justin. After she fed and changed him, she placed him in his bassinet. Almost immediately, she began shaking uncontrollably. She picked up the phone but was shaking so bad, she had trouble dialing 9-1-1. As strange as it may seem, she was able to dial my mother's 10-digit phone number. I have to believe it was meant to go that way. That is how God works! I had been a nervous wreck, but God was moving in the situation from the very beginning.

As the hours passed, I received more details about the situation. By the time the paramedics arrived, Yashica, who did manage to crawl to the door, had a pulse rate in the 20's. A normal pulse rate for a woman is approximately 72 – 80 beats per minute. For adults, a temperature of 100° Fahrenheit indicates a fever. Yashica's temperature at the time the paramedics arrived was 105° Fahrenheit. With a pulse rate in the 20's and a temperature of 105°, my sister was staring death in the face. After assessing her condition, the paramedics worked on Yashica before transporting her to the same hospital where she had given birth just days before. It was truly the grace of God that kept her alive that night.

For the next three weeks, Yashica lay in the hospital while doctors and specialists came and went, telling her very little about her condition. In fact, the only thing they seemed to be able to surmise was that she had some type of infection. An infection? What type of infection? What brought it on? Were there any signs of infection before she was released from the hospital? How were they planning to treat this infection? There had to be *something* they could tell us. What was even more strange was the fact that Yashica's doctor, who didn't seem quite sure about her condition, wanted to operate on her. At that point, we began to wonder if something had been left inside her during the cesarean delivery. My mother, who had been caring for Justin during Yashica's hospital stay, was becoming increasingly agitated. The only thing we seemed to know with any degree of certainty was that Yashica was very near death during the early morning hours of August 2nd, and we didn't even really know why.

About a month and a half after this horrendous ordeal, Yashica was visiting with us in Savannah when she asked if she could speak to me alone. During this weighty conversation, she informed me that she had gone to see another doctor. This new doctor, having reviewed her case, determined she needed to test Yashica for ovarian cancer.

"Cancer?" I asked as if I didn't hear her correctly.

"Yeah. She just wants to rule it out. There's nothing to worry about."

"But there has to be some reason she thinks this might be what's wrong with you."

"Stacy, she just wants to rule it out. It's no big deal."

Yashica sounded so sure that it was *no big deal*. As I began to launch my own, personal prayer crusade on her behalf, I realized that a year and a half had passed since I gave birth to Angel. Getting pregnant had never been a problem for me. It was *staying* pregnant that had proven to be the challenge. With that in mind, I made an appointment with Dr. Robinson. After all, it was time for a routine pap smear. With everything that had been going on, I hadn't even realized that I had not had one confirmed pregnancy in over a year.

"So, can you think of any reason I have not gotten pregnant yet?" I asked almost immediately after my pap smear.

"Well," Dr. Robinson began, "there could be a number of reasons. Here's what we'll do. It's September now. Let's get through the holidays and if nothing happens by January, we'll do a laparoscopy so I can take a look and see what's going on."

That seemed fair enough for me. I left the doctor's office feeling pretty good about that plan. I could spend the next few months focusing on my family. I just wanted to enjoy that time. While we had not heard word on Yashica's diagnosis yet, we were elated to still have her with us. We just needed time not to worry about illness or infertility. We needed to focus on something positive.

Our focus shifted swiftly, however, with a devastating piece of news. We learned in mid-October that Yashica did, in fact, have ovarian cancer. The one silver lining was that she was given a positive prognosis. Her doctor indicated that the disease had been detected early enough that it could be treated with radiation and possibly surgery. At this juncture, she did not believe chemotherapy would be necessary. Regardless of the prognosis, this was a very tough pill to swallow. I had been trying for three years to have a baby. As if that wasn't enough of a blow to my faith walk, my 25-year-old sister had now been diagnosed with the silent killer that is ovarian cancer.

It was becoming increasingly more difficult to understand God's plan. I could not grasp what He was doing or where He was taking us, but I knew I could not get there without a show of faith. I had to keep believing. I had to keep trusting. I had to keep the faith…for Yashica *and* for me.

CHAPTER EIGHT

New Assignment... New Calling

With my sister's cancer diagnosis and my realization that it had been nearly two years since my last pregnancy, I was at a spiritual crossroads. I often felt helpless and could not fathom that anyone would understand the gravity of my situation. Based on my teachings, I was supposed to endure and begin to praise God for what He was going to do. The Bible tells us that faith comes by hearing, and I was definitely hearing. Attending church had become a major priority for me. I attended worship service on Sundays and bible study on Wednesday evenings. I was a copious note taker, ensuring that I didn't miss any vital points of the messages.

I was clearly growing spiritually, and I was fully aware that life would not be without trials and my share of burdens to bear. The heavier my burden became, however, the more inadequate I felt to carry it. Not only did I consider how badly I wanted to become a mother, but I considered the role I played in preventing Jerome from becoming a father. What a harsh reality to face! He might never know the joys of fatherhood because of my body's shortcomings. It just seemed so unfair.

As if the load wasn't heavy enough, I had the onerous task of being there for my sister. I almost felt undeserving of the role I was now playing in her life. How could I encourage her to trust in God and have faith that she would be healed when my faith was being tested on so many levels? There was something in the depth of my spirit that told me that I would be able to do this. I just had to remember that the faith that God was building in me would have to be strong enough to move mountains. Mountain-moving faith doesn't come by way of wimpy trials. I had to *really* go through something!

Yashica began her radiation treatments in early November with very little side effects. Although I had tasked myself with encouraging her, I found myself being encouraged by the amazing strength she exuded. I wasn't sure if she was that strong or if she was playing the same song-and-dance I had been playing regarding my infertility. Regardless of her intentions, I think maintaining a positive outlook was paramount to her healing process. We were both in the fights of our lives, and I realized that we were both ultimately fighting for the same thing – our babies. She was fighting to be here to raise hers, and I was fighting to get mine here so I could raise them.

"Tribulation worketh patience; and patience, experience; and experience, hope." There were these words again, echoing in my spirit.

I knew I needed to develop my patience in order to strengthen my faith. Faith requires us to believe in something we don't see, and that takes strength. It was a process, and I still had a ways to go. The funny thing is I might not have realized that had I not faced this challenge. I just always believed my faith was strong. That was until it was truly tested. I just kept telling myself that everything would be okay. Although my faith wasn't quite where it needed to be, I somehow felt that everything was going to be okay. God had not forgotten about me, His servant, had He?

As January approached, I gave careful thought to what Dr. Robinson had said. If I had not conceived, I would need to see him to schedule a laparoscopy. This procedure would involve Dr. Robinson making a small incision in my naval and inserting a tiny camera that would allow him to see directly into my pelvic cavity. What he would find would hopefully be the answer to the question of why I had not conceived in two years.

Having met with Dr. Robinson, my surgery was scheduled for January 26, 2006. I was excited and scared all at the same time. I was excited because I felt this represented a positive step in my fertility treatment. However, I was afraid of what the procedure might reveal. All I could do was pray for a positive outcome.

It was a beautiful, peaceful Sunday morning about one week before my surgery. Yashica happened to be in town and wanted to attend church with Jerome and me. We opted to attend the 8:00a.m. service on this particular day. Yashica had progressed well in her treatment and would soon be finished. The next step in her treatment would likely include tests to ensure the cancer had not spread to any other organs and removal of the affected ovary. God was moving in her situation in a miraculous way. She was being healed right before my eyes. I was ashamed that I was so afraid for my own health after seeing what He was doing for my sister. All the literature I found on ovarian cancer talked about five-year survival rates. That's how deadly this disease is. It is almost as if it is unrealistic to expect to live beyond five years. I was determined that my sister would live many years beyond her diagnosis. God is greater than any doctor's report we could receive. My sister *would* beat this! Now, it was time for me to incorporate that same fervor in believing that my womb would be healed.

We selected a pew towards the middle of the church and took our seats. What began as an ordinary worship service would turn out to be a day we would not soon forget. Shortly before Bishop Odum began his sermon, he went up and stood behind his book board. The sanctuary was virtually silent as the congregation awaited his next statement. He scanned the congregation and then looked back down at his book board. I think it was apparent to everyone that he had something to say. As he scanned the congregation a second time, he finally spoke. What he said caught me completely off guard.

"Brother Stanton, please stand."

As I looked over at Jerome, he appeared as though he wasn't sure Bishop Odum meant to say his name. Nonetheless, he slowly stood to his feet.

"Brother Stanton is a quiet man," Bishop Odum continued. "If you didn't see him, you wouldn't know he was here. He has a quiet strength about him. Brother Stanton, would you be willing to work in your church?"

In a strong, sure voice, Jerome declared, "Yes, Sir."

Bishop Odum looked over at Deacon Richardson, who chaired the Deacons' Ministry at that time, and asked him to escort Jerome to the deacons' section. As Deacon Richardson made his way down the aisle, the congregation exploded in applause. I wiped the lone tear that tried to escape the corner of my eye. As I watched my husband take his place among the deacons, I thought of that quiet strength

Bishop Odum had spoken of and how pivotal it had been during our challenges with infertility.

As the congregation settled down, Bishop Odum rendered another surprise. He glanced over at Jerome with a smile.

"Now, Brother Stanton, go back and get your wife."

As the congregation burst into another round of applause, Jerome made his way down the aisle and took me by the hand. We walked, hand in hand, down the aisle and took our seats. I was overcome with emotion. I was happy. I was nervous. I was surprised, to say the least. Was this what I thought it was? Jerome and I, being called to the office of deacon? This was such a tall order. While our primary goal was to serve God, we knew so little about the proper way to serve in this capacity. I thought of the challenges I had been facing and how my faith was questionable at best. Bishop Odum pointed out something very profound about what had just taken place. He does not call anyone to the office of deacon whom God has not revealed to him as a servant in this capacity.

This was even more puzzling. God had revealed to Bishop Odum that *I* should be called to the office of deacon? God is omniscient, so He was well aware of the struggles I had been having with my faith walk. As a deacon, I would need to be strong in my faith and able to be a steadfast witness for God. I would need to be attuned to my relationship with God. While I was honored to have been chosen, I was not completely confident that I was ready to serve. Ready or not, I had been called of God.

I knew that it was my responsibility to heed the call, but I also knew I needed direction from God. By all accounts, there was nothing special about me. I was a young woman who loved God and who had made the claim that I knew Him for myself. I was also a young woman who was in the middle of a storm – a storm that had caused me to question God and to further question my faith in Him. So, what made me fit to serve as a deacon? The word of God tells us:

Likewise must deacons be grave, not double-tongued, not given to much wine, not greedy of filthy lucre; Holding the mystery of the faith in a pure conscience. And let these also first be proved; then let them use the office of a deacon, being found blameless.

For they that have used the office of a deacon well purchase to themselves a good degree, and great boldness in the faith which is in Christ Jesus. (I Timothy 3:8-10,13)

As I thought on this passage of scripture, my mind became fixed on the statement, "And let these also first be proved..." Maybe this was the very answer to my questions regarding my tottering faith. I needed to be tested. I needed to prove to God that I was a sincere servant. How can faith that has not been tested truly be affirmed? Maybe it was all a part of God's plan to take the very thing I so desired and use it to test the limits of my faith. Until this revelation, I had not done so well in this test. I had allowed myself to be easily discouraged and to question God. I allowed myself to nearly give up. God could not use me in that place. He needed me to be sure of my faith. Moreover, He needed me to understand that when the blessing I had been praying for was fully manifested, He should receive all of the glory. To that end, the tests became more rigorous.

On January 26, 2006, I reported to Memorial Health University Medical Center around 6:00a.m. for my laparoscopy. Having completed pre-op paperwork the previous day, my admissions process ensued rather smoothly. To await my procedure, I was placed in a small room, about the size of an examination room in a doctor's office. Shortly after I arrived, a nurse came in to start my IV, and an anesthesiologist came in to explain the process and risks involved in being put to sleep. He also administered a mild sedative. Being no stranger to surgery, this was all very routine to me. I was even given a pregnancy test.

At the appropriate time, I left Jerome in the small room and was wheeled into a very cold operating room. The lights were blinding. I lay there, staring at the ceiling as I awaited the anesthesiologist. As Dr. Robinson began to prepare, a nurse walked into the room and whispered something to him and the other staff that was present. The activity about the room came to a crashing halt. Needless to say, I was very confused by this and a little anxious. I could hear Dr. Robinson asking the staff to wheel me back to the small holding room. What on earth was going on?

I would soon find out that something very peculiar had transpired. It seems that the pregnancy test I had been administered rendered a negative result, but as it sat on the counter, the reading began to appear positive. Because of this, it was determined that the test was inconclusive.

Dr. Robinson explained to me that he had ordered a blood test to determine whether I was in fact pregnant. If the test returned a positive result, the surgery would obviously be cancelled. I sat there in complete awe of this situation. A pregnancy test renders a positive result when the pregnancy hormone has been detected. So, how does a test go from negative to positive? The only plausible explanation was that if I was pregnant, it could have been so early that the hormone level was extremely low.

The blood test rendered a negative result, and the surgery ensued. As I awoke in the recovery room, a nurse explained to me that there had been no complications and that I would be given time to rest and would be released that afternoon. I was taken to another of those small rooms and allowed to rest. I felt incredibly groggy and lethargic. I was not quite sure how long I had slept, but I awoke with this overwhelming feeling of nausea. As I glanced about the room, my eyes caught Jerome's. He was sitting next to my bed, looking as if he had been studying me as I slept.

"Hey," he said, rubbing his hand across my face.

"Hey," I responded, "have you talked to Dr. Robinson yet?"

"Briefly."

Although I was not completely alert, I got the feeling Jerome was trying to avoid the conversation I was so eager to have.

"Did he tell you anything?" I insisted.

"He showed me pictures of your organs," he started slowly.

"Well?"

"He showed me your uterus, your ovaries, and your fallopian tubes. He said something about a complete blockage, but he said we're a young couple and could probably do in-vitro."

At that moment, I felt my throat tightening. Jerome sounded as if he had rehearsed how he would say this to me. I felt as though I could not breathe. I began to vomit, but the only thing that came up was water. Jerome quickly summoned a nurse, who tried to get me to eat crackers. I didn't want any crackers. I didn't want any ginger ale. I just wanted to go back to sleep. If this was the best news I could receive, I would rather have gone back to sleep. The small room seemed to be getting even smaller. Faith. Patience. Deacon. Proven. Perfect Plan. My mind was racing, and I began to cry. As quickly as the tears flowed, Jerome wiped them. I wanted to see Dr. Robinson. I needed to hear this from him. I was so hoping Jerome had misconstrued some part of the message. The next morning, as I was resting at home, the phone rang.

"Hello," I said, still a little groggy.

"Hello, Stacy?"

"Yes."

"Dr. Robinson here. I know I'm supposed to see you for a follow-up next week, but I wanted to talk to you about something. I wanted to make sure you understand what is happening."

"Okay."

"Well, I think we have figured out why you haven't gotten pregnant since your last loss."

I listened in silence.

"As I performed the laparoscopic procedure, I placed dye in both your fallopian tubes. It flowed to a certain point and stopped, which indicates a blockage. It appears there are blockages in both your tubes right at the point where they meet the ovaries. This could have possibly been caused by scar tissue that may have developed following a previous surgery."

"So now what?" I kept my statements short and simple.

Being the eternal optimist, Dr. Robinson tried to get me to embrace what he thought was a silver lining.

"We can still get a baby. We just have to be a little more creative. We have to bypass the blockage, and this can be done through in vitro fertilization. During this procedure, the egg is taken from your ovary, fertilized in a lab and placed into your uterus."

This was too much for me to process. I just sat there, holding the phone. Not knowing what to say next, I just uttered, "So, if the procedure is successful, will you be my doctor during the pregnancy?"

"Yes, I will."

"Okay." I wanted Dr. Robinson to think I saw this as good news.

My mother, who had been at the hospital when this news was delivered to Jerome, tried to comfort me as best she could. She could not believe that after three failed pregnancies, I was now unable to conceive naturally. Both she and Yashica tried to put a positive spin on in vitro fertilization. The truth of the matter, though, was that this procedure involved so much more than the procedure itself. Before undergoing the procedure, I would have to take hormones to ensure I produced a large number of eggs. Several eggs would be removed from my ovaries and fertilized. The fertilized eggs would be placed into my uterus in hopes that at least one of them would implant. *If* the procedure was successful, all would be well, but if not, we would have to repeat the *cycle*. In vitro fertilization could cost nearly $20,000 and is not covered by most insurance plans. It is also not guaranteed.

As Jerome and I sat in the doctor's office a week later, this new hurdle became even more real to me. Dr. Robinson showed me pictures to support what he had told Jerome and me. There my fallopian tubes were, in living color. Blocked. It was real. No matter how I tried to spin this scenario in my mind, it was real. I had suffered two miscarriages and the loss of a premature newborn only to learn almost two years later that my fallopian tubes were completely blocked. Both of them. Blocked. It was like a garden hose folded over to stop the flow of water. Dr. Robinson even used a diagram that was hanging on the wall to show me exactly where the blockages were.

Just as the room began to close in on me in much the same way it had in the hospital, my dear husband spoke.

"Have you ever heard of anyone's tubes opening up on their own?"

Dr. Robinson and I glanced over at Jerome, and I couldn't help smiling. As I listened to Jerome's words, I could also hear, "holding the mystery of the faith in a pure conscience," and "let these also first be proved." As I waited to hear Dr. Robinson's response to Jerome's question, I became amazingly calm. Amazingly peaceful. I was finally getting it. I was finally starting to understand that every let-down had been God's way of building us up to fulfill a greater purpose. It was finally becoming clear.

Dr. Robinson proceeded to tell us that he had heard of anecdotes and stories of tubes opening up, but he didn't want me building any false hope. Dr. Robinson was nothing if not honest. He went on to tell us of a very reputable reproductive endocrinologist, or fertility specialist, who had a very high success rate helping infertile couples realize their dreams of parenthood. This was the same doctor who had accompanied Dr. Robinson during my myomectomy. We reluctantly agreed to see him.

Dr. Robinson had his staff make the appointment for me before we left, explaining that this doctor was usually booked months in advance. We managed to get an appointment for March 3, 2006. This date would mark two years since I had given birth to and lost Angel. Wow! On Angel's birthday, we would be meeting with the doctor who could possibly help us give her a sibling.

CHAPTER NINE

Turning Point

Despite what I had learned after my laparoscopy, I was at a surprisingly peaceful place. It was as though my spirit would not allow me to accept that this was the final call. I began to thoroughly examine the whole issue of faith. As we are told in Hebrews 11:1, *Now faith is the substance of things hoped for, the evidence of things not seen.*

Throughout this entire experience, I believe I failed most at being consistent in my faith walk. Each time my situation appeared to be getting better, my faith seemed to grow stronger. Quite the opposite was true whenever there was a setback. I was gradually beginning to realize that drawing closer to God and trying to better understand what He required of me would be the key to overcoming this storm.

To demonstrate to God that I fully trusted Him, I had to exhibit faith even when the forecast was grim. It is impossible to please God without faith, so it became imperative that I shifted my focus from questioning God and feeling sorry for myself to praising Him even for the things hoped for and the things not seen. It seemed that ever since Jerome posed the question to Dr. Robinson regarding the fallopian tubes opening up, a sense of serenity came over me. I was no longer anxious about my situation. I was excited more than anything about what God was going to do. The way I prayed about the situation was even starting to change. It was no longer about asking God to allow me to conceive. It was about me asking God to prepare me to receive the blessing in His time.

Because I was pretty certain that I would be emotionally drained, I took a sick day on Friday, March 3, 2006. It could be 20 years after

Angel's demise, and I would think of her on that date. I had resolved that she would always be a very special part of me. Somehow, I always feel close to her, and I felt she knew me even though she never opened her eyes to look into my face.

As we exited the elevator, I took a deep breath. This was it. We were on our way to visit a highly reputable fertility specialist. Jerome placed his arm around me and assured me that everything would be okay. He reminded me that we were in this together.

As I scanned the waiting room, I began to feel so sad. I didn't feel sad for myself as much as I felt sad about the reality that so many women were facing infertility. I did not know the specific plight of each woman there, but I did know that each woman's visit came on the heels of the revelation that she could not naturally bear children. I silently prayed that we would all get what we came there for.

"Stacy Stanton," a young lady in scrubs stood at the door, calling for me.

Jerome and I followed her to a back office where she ascertained our personal information and made a copy of our insurance card. She explained to us that while they do file claims with insurance companies as a courtesy, many fertility treatments are not covered. What she did next was extremely puzzling. She took a photo of Jerome and me and placed it in our file. She then told us that we would be called in to see the doctor in just a few moments.

As we walked into the doctor's office, I remember thinking that he must have been helping many families realize their dreams of parenthood. His office was very plush. He sat behind a cherry desk in a large, leather chair. We took our seats directly in front of his desk in comfortable leather chairs. After we got past the introductions, the fertility specialist took out a pen and yellow legal pad. He then looked directly at me.

"Okay, I want you to tell me your story from the very beginning."

Was he joking? He *had* to be joking. It was Angel's birthday, which made this visit difficult enough. Now, I was tasked with providing this man with a somewhat stoic demeanor a play-by-play account of everything I had gone through.

With Jerome holding my hand, I managed to get through every painful detail of my struggle with infertility. I told of the miscarriages I had had in October 2002 and July 2003. I told of my pregnancy with Angel and how it ended abruptly with an emergency cesarean delivery 16 weeks prior to her due date. I told of her death shortly after her birth and ended my synopsis with news of the recent revelation that my fallopian tubes were blocked, possibly due to scar tissue. As painful as this was, I was proud of myself for getting through it without shedding one tear.

At each juncture, the fertility specialist appeared to be taking copious notes. He listened attentively, but showed no emotion. While my story was unique to me, he had probably met many *Stacy Stantons* during his career. He rarely looked up from his notepad. He just kept nodding.

It wasn't until he began to speak that this consultation became extremely uncomfortable. He placed his ink pen on top of his legal pad and looked directly at me.

"Well, the first thing I would like to do is perform a procedure to confirm the blockage in your tubes. This procedure, known as a hysterosalpingogram, or HSG, will involve me forcing dye through both your fallopian tubes. There will be some cramping and discomfort, but the procedure will only last a few seconds. This will allow me to determine if your tubes are completely blocked. If they are blocked, we have two options, a tubioplasty or in vitro fertilization."

Although he did not exude the same compassionate demeanor I had grown accustomed to with Dr. Robinson, I still wanted to hear what he had to say, at least at that moment. As it turned out, the more he had to say, the less I wanted to hear. Jerome and I sat in complete disbelief at some of the things this man said.

He started by suggesting that if I were to become pregnant, I would have to be hung up by my toes in order to hold the fetus in place. Maybe he meant it as a joke, but unfortunately, our bout with infertility was no joke to us. Perhaps he was so accustomed to seeing patients who were facing infertility that he became desensitized. Perhaps he had a *God* complex. After hearing what this man had to say, I was eager to let him know that I served a God who was more than capable of turning my situation around in His time and in His way. When the fertility specialist suggested that one of our sisters carried our baby for us, we knew the visit was over. Maybe I was not in the right frame of mind to receive any of what the specialist said, or maybe it was at that moment that I truly realized where my help comes from.

I had no problem with this man being honest with us, but it was the brutal, uncompassionate manner with which he delivered his message. Most patients who visit his office are probably in a place of desperation. We were anything but desperate. Prior to our departure, the specialist asked us to stop by the receptionist's desk to make an appointment for my HSG. We walked right past the receptionist's desk and out the door.

As we stepped onto the elevator, tears began to roll down my face. Jerome wrapped his arms around me and asked, "You didn't receive that, did you?"

"No," I said through my sea of tears.

That day, on that elevator, we prayed together and vowed to leave this situation in God's hands once and for all. God was the ultimate healer. He was the ultimate fertility specialist. It was truly time to trust His plan. We were not sure what our next step needed to be, but we were sure that we had seen the last of the fertility specialist.

Upon our arrival at our home, I was met with a pleasant surprise. I retrieved the mail and noticed there was a card addressed to me. The card had come from my friend, Lisa. She had sent it in an effort to let me know she was thinking of me on Angel's birthday. Also thinking of me was my friend, Kisha, whose son's birthday was also March 3rd. It meant so much to me for her to think of my aching heart on her son's birthday. These ladies probably never fully understood what their gestures meant to me.

The interesting thing about the tribulations I had endured was that I had to realize that it was my cross to bear. While people sympathize with you, it's important to understand that the grieving period may extend beyond the sympathetic period. I believe it is just human nature. Tragedies happen. Those affected grieve. Those close to those affected sympathize. Eventually, life goes on. Having endured other tragedies in my life, I had come to understand this process far too well. To that end, I never expected much fanfare on Angel's birthday. So, to have someone remember year after year meant so much.

Although the day was emotionally draining, I was extremely happy to have mental clarity. It was as if I needed that meeting with the fertility specialist in order to move on. I could no longer remain on the proverbial fence. I had two very succinct choices. I could trust God's plan, or I could drown in self-pity and give up. In that doctor's office, I had made a choice. I chose to trust the promise of God. What a way to celebrate Angel's birthday!

One day, shortly after Angel's birthday, I happened to be at home alone. Feeling the need to truly connect with God, I took this opportunity to pray. I knelt beside my bed and buried my face in my cupped hands. As I closed my eyes tightly, I reflected over the heartache. I reflected over the pain. I reflected on the hope. I reflected on the feelings of inadequacy. In this quiet place, in this tranquil moment, I began to speak to God.

> *Father, in the name of Jesus, I kneel before you.*
> *I come before your throne in the spirit of humility and thanksgiving.*
> *I am so grateful to you today, God. I know I would be nothing without you, and I come*
> *before you, just offering up my gratitude. Lord, it's no secret that the past few years*
> *have been difficult for me. I have hurt. Lord, I have cried.*
> *I have felt so very low, but, Lord, you kept me.*
> *You kept me when Satan tried to plant seeds of suicide in my mind.*
> *You kept me when I was alone in my mother's house, suffering a miscarriage!*
> *Lord, you are so worthy of my praise, and I love you so much.*
> *I owe you everything! I owe my life to you, God!*
> *Lord, I know I have not always lived in a way that pleased you, but*
> *it is by your grace that I am able to be in a better place.*
> *I need to feel your presence. I need to be close to you, God.*
> *I need you like I've never needed anything or anyone before.*
> *This is a prayer of expectancy. I am expecting you to move in my situation.*
> *Lord, I can't finish the race without you. I realize now that I must trust your plan.*
> *Lord, I want to thank you for Jerome and for his strength. I want to thank you*
> *for all the friends and family who have interceded on my behalf.*
> *I thank you, Lord, for not leaving me! Lord, I thank you! Lord, I thank you!*
> *I am nothing without you! I thank you! Lord, I am no longer*
> *asking that you allow me to become pregnant. Rather than your permissive will, Lord,*
> *I want to see your perfect will manifested in my life.*
> *I don't want to do this my way, Lord!*

I want to do this your way, God!
Lord, when I gave birth to Angel, you saw fit to spare my life.
God, I know you are not finished with me.
I know you still have work for me to do.
I surrender to you, God! I stretch my hands to you, God!
I want to do it your way, God! I love you so much, Lord!
I am so sorry! Lord, I am so sorry for doubting you! I'm so sorry!
I'm so sorry for questioning you! I am so sorry for not being everything you would have me be. I want to live for you, God! I want you to get the glory in all I do.
It's in your hands! Let your will be done.
Yes, I want to be a mother, but, Lord, I want to do it your way and in your time. Lord, if it's your will to bless me with a child, I will love that child and
teach him to have a reverent fear of you. Let your will be done.
Lord, please give me strength! Please give me strength to accept your plan for my life. Lord, I thank you. I thank you for what you have done and for what you will do!
I thank you for the blood that saved me! I thank you for mercy!
I thank you for your grace! I thank you, Lord!
I just want to feel your presence in my life. I want to hear from you, God!
I love you, I thank you, and I give you the glory. In Jesus's name, I pray. Amen.

As I closed my prayer, my hands were no longer cupped. They were stretched across my bed, and my face was covered with tears. I could barely move, so I sat there, crying. I finally conjured up enough energy to get up. This sealed it. What had taken place in the elevator after leaving the fertility specialist was further sealed by my prayer. I could move forward now. Having relinquished my situation to God and trusting the plan He had for my life, I could face the challenges that would come. I can do all things through Christ who strengthens me (Philippians 4:13). It was done. All I had to do now was believe.

CHAPTER TEN

Revelation

One of my favorite gospel artists is Smokie Norful. When I hear his music, I don't get the feeling I'm listening to an average run-of-the-mill gospel artist who's just trying to sell records. I am listening to a storyteller. I am listening to a child of God who does not mind becoming transparent enough to share his testimony. He is a true witness for God.

I can vividly remember one day about a month after our visit with the fertility specialist. I was in my car, and my thoughts somehow turned to Angel. I even thought of the babies I never got to name. I thought of my sister and what she was going through. This was one of those days I needed God to strengthen me the way I had asked Him to in that pivotal prayer beside my bed. Our team was gearing up for WalkAmerica 2006, but on this particular day, I wasn't very excited about that or anything else. I was in a somewhat somber mood.

As I drove along, a song came on the radio that almost made me pull over. It was absolutely beautiful, and the words spoke right to my heart. The song was titled *I Understand*, and the artist was none other than Mr. Smokie Norful. The song was written in God's voice, and He was imploring the listener to trust His plan. He was saying to wait one more day and one more step. In the song, God wants the listener to know that He sees what he or she has been going through, and He does understand.

As I pulled into my driveway, I rested my head on the steering wheel and continued to listen to Smokie. While listening, it began to seem as though I was no longer hearing Smokie's voice, but the quiet, still voice of God. I sat there with my head planted firmly on the steering wheel, listening.

Stacy, I've seen everything you've gone through.
When you became discouraged and questioned me, I forgave you.
I forgave you because I knew when I set this plan in motion,
it would be difficult for you.
I also knew how much you could bear.
I knew even before I created you in your mother's womb.
I knew even then that you would go through this test of your faith.
Stacy, I need you to trust my plan. I see you. I hear your cries.
I know everything about you. I know the desires of your heart.
Think over your life, my child.
When have I ever left you? When have I ever forsaken you?
Of course there have been some trials, but how can you truly
follow the path I have set for your life if you don't have a testimony?
I know the road seems long, but you mustn't grow weary.
You have said you felt your faith was weak.
Well, my child, every time you rejoiced with a friend who had a healthy baby,
you demonstrated faith. When you were there during your sister's pregnancy,
you demonstrated faith. Every time you cared for someone else's child,
you demonstrated faith. Every time you offered encouragement to
other women facing infertility, you demonstrated faith.
Your involvement with the March of Dimes cause was a
demonstration of faith. My child, nothing in your life has been a mistake.
The path you have traveled has been by design.
You were chosen. You are so special to me.
I understand. Just hold on a little while longer. Just hold on. I am God.
Your journey will not be in vain.
Please realize that if I had manifested the blessing before you were ready to
receive it, I might not have gotten the glory.
Now, when you see a shift in your situation,
you will know it was me.

As I raised my head from the steering wheel, I felt totally rejuvenated. No, God did not sit down in the passenger seat of my car and speak to me, but He spoke into my spirit. I was at peace. There was nothing else for me to do but await the manifestation.

Easter was quickly approaching, and I was looking forward to the worship experience. I was also looking forward to watching my brother and nephew recite their speeches. Yashica was planning a trip to Savannah for the Easter holiday. Even with the excitement surrounding the impending holiday, I could not discount the peculiar discomfort I was beginning to experience.

For the entire week that preceded Easter, I felt a little strange. True to form, I attempted to ignore the subtle signs my body was giving. On April 8, 2006, I conducted a 6-hour job readiness workshop for high school students from across the state. Upon returning home that evening, I felt terrible. My energy was low, I was experiencing cramping, and I even noticed some spotting. I minimized all of this by attributing the feelings to being on my feet all day.

As the week progressed, the cramping slightly increased in intensity. I can recall being out with my mother on Thursday of that week. We did a little shopping and ate all the wrong foods. I even stopped at one of my favorite smoothie shops for a strawberry smoothie. Later that night, I found myself in the bathroom, vomiting. The very next day, I decided to go out on a limb and take a home pregnancy test. Sure, I was still keenly aware of my blocked tubes, but I had nothing to lose by just taking a test. I could not believe what I saw! It was positive!

Still experiencing spotting and cramping, I continued to prepare for Easter service. The doctor's office was closed, so I decided to just try and enjoy my weekend and worry about it on Monday. With the exception of Jerome, I opted not to tell anyone about the positive test. Throughout the weekend, I took two more tests, both of which yielded positive results.

On Easter Sunday afternoon, my family joined us at our home for dinner. My spotting had increased to a light menstrual-like flow. As we enjoyed our family time on this sacred holiday, I decided to speak to Yashica privately. I called her into my room and showed her the three pregnancy tests I had taken. She was completely in awe. I explained to Yashica that the reason I wanted her to see these was because I wanted to encourage her.

I admitted to her that the spotting, the cramping, and eventually the bleeding were likely indications that I was having a miscarriage. I wanted her to understand that I would be okay either way because I was the young lady who was not supposed to be able to conceive. I had pictures of my blocked fallopian tubes. I had tangible, irrefutable proof that I had a blockage in both tubes. So, miscarriage or not, a positive pregnancy test just confirmed what God had already spoken into my spirit. I wanted Yashica to be encouraged in her battle with cancer. I wanted her to know that I believed we were both on the verge of a breakthrough. For the first time, I knew we would both be healed.

By Monday, the bleeding was a little heavier and the cramping was much worse. I contacted Dr. Robinson's office so I could learn something more conclusive. My pregnancy test initially appeared negative, and I explained to the nurse that I had gotten three positive tests at home over the weekend. Dr. Robinson ordered a blood test, which rendered a positive result. He explained to me that the hormone level usually doubled daily in the early weeks of pregnancy. He further explained that a decrease in the hormone level usually signified an impending miscarriage. I was asked to return to the office on Wednesday for a second blood test to assess the hormone level.

As I had expected, the second test indicated a significant drop in the hormone level. So, on April 19, 2006, I suffered the loss of my fourth confirmed pregnancy. To some, this might seem incredibly tragic, but I had a somewhat different perspective. While it was not my wish to suffer through anymore miscarriages, I realized that a miscarriage could not have occurred without conception. Just three months prior, I had been told and given tangible evidence that natural conception was no longer possible due to blockages in my fallopian tubes.

I had looked on as my husband asked my doctor if he had heard of anyone's tubes becoming *unblocked* on their own. I had stood in an elevator after a very uncomfortable visit with a fertility specialist and prayed with my husband. I had prayed privately, surrendering this whole situation to God. I had sat in my car as God spoke into my spirit regarding His plan for my life. Now, on April 19th, I was suffering a miscarriage. To me, this miscarriage represented a turning point in my situation. I was never administered any fertility treatments of any kind. By all accounts, my womb was barren, but God was clearly demonstrating to me what He had spoken in my spirit.

He said He would never leave nor forsake me. He said if I just trusted His plan, He would begin to move in my situation. Jerome and I both knew what we had seen on the pictures. The blockages in my tubes were real. Yet, I was able to conceive with no medical help. How could I not give God the glory in that? This was but a small indication of the way in which God was getting ready to move in my life. Just as Easter represented the resurrection of Jesus Christ, this miscarriage represented the resurrection of my fertility.

Approximately two weeks after Easter, I got a phone call from a college friend. She was calling to announce that she and her husband were expecting their first child. Although I was extremely happy for her, I couldn't help wondering why she had waited 15 weeks into her pregnancy to share her news with me. When I hung up the phone, it became crystal clear. She was slow to share her news because she was concerned what affect it might have on me. While I know that she meant well, I was somewhat unnerved.

Upon hanging up the phone with my friend, I realized something. Throughout my ordeal, I had been reduced to a fragile person who needed to be protected from the cycle of life that was going on all around me. Maybe I had worn my feelings on my sleeve, or maybe it was inconceivable how someone could be experiencing such a trying ordeal and still be okay. I would be the first to admit that there were moments when I did appear not be handling my situation well.

I believe it is human nature to analyze people and their problems. I had been told that Jerome and I should consider adoption. I had even been told that I might have overreacted to my consultation with the fertility specialist. I was told that my refusal to accept fertility treatments indicated that I was giving up. I was given a myriad of unsolicited advice. I think people's reactions ranged from pity to protection. Some even thought I was causing undue stress on Jerome and me by continuing to try for a baby. Although the fertility specialist came across crass and uncompassionate, I was told he was just doing his job. It was rarely, "Stacy, how do you feel?" More often, it was, "Stacy, maybe you should just do this or maybe you can't handle that."

It was amazing because the more people assessed my situation, the more I sought God. The more I felt I could not handle the situation, the more He showed me *He* could. It was only His voice I needed to hear. I admit I didn't realize this when my trials began, but I knew now that I did not need pity. I did not need advice I had not asked for. I did not need to be protected. I was chosen of God. He knew from the very first miscarriage how my story would unfold. In order to truly be a witness for Him, I had to go through this process. It was in this storm that I felt the presence of God in a way I had not all my life. The way I saw it, I was better off than most.

CHAPTER ELEVEN

The Prophecy

Our team, Earth Angels, was phenomenally successful in our second year of participation in the March of Dimes' WalkAmerica event. The event took place on April 29, 2006, and our team of more than 40 walkers raised more than $6,000. With the exception of four corporate teams, we raised more money than all other teams in the Coastal Empire. I could not have been more proud. In our daughter's name, we had made significant strides in the fight against prematurity and infant mortality.

During the post-walk festivities, the executive director of the local March of Dimes chapter introduced me to a young lady who had lost her baby to prematurity approximately one month prior. As the young lady began to cry, I embraced her. Remembering my emotional state one month after losing Angel, I tried as best I could to encourage this young mother. I knew too well that disheartening feeling of being a mother but having no child to show for it. This young lady, a complete stranger, cried on my shoulder as if she had known me all her life. I looked her square in the eye and declared to her that God is faithful and that her baby would always be a part of her spirit. What I really wanted to convey to her was that she would get through this.

Through her river of tears, she managed to thank me. What meant more was that she seemed to embrace what I had said about God being faithful. I knew it was a possibility that I may never see this young lady again, but I felt I had encouraged her in some small way. I was so pleased that I was able to take such a gratifying leap in the right direction.

With the walk behind me, I shifted my focus to my sister-in-law's impending wedding. This was a very exciting *and* stressful time for her, and as her matron of honor, I made a concerted effort to assist her in any way I could. It was nice to be so heavily involved in something that didn't remind me of my losses.

I found that I was finally in a place where I was not sulking as much. As I awaited a move from God, I was busy with the affairs of life. It had been so long since I had such an immense feeling of peace. I had endured a few bumps and bruises, but I was still in the race. I had developed this quiet strength that forced me to face my situation head on. I was no longer afraid. I was no longer fragile. For the first time in approximately four years, I was in a great spiritual, emotional, and mental place. I'm not saying I didn't have some challenging days, but I was much better equipped to handle them.

I was elated by the news my family received in early May. To add strength to my newfound peace, we received word that Yashica had been officially declared cancer-free. While she still faced surgery, this was a major feat. As with my situation, I knew that God must get the glory. I could not help thinking of the first lady of the Civil Rights movement, Mrs. Coretta Scott King, who had died in January 2006 after being diagnosed with ovarian cancer in November 2005. Ovarian cancer is detected early in only 20% of its sufferers, so to have my sister receive an early diagnosis and be able to be treated with radiation was simply by the grace of God.

As I witnessed God at work, I was beginning to realize that His perfect will superseded what doctors said or what we sometimes allowed ourselves to believe. God was showing His faithfulness and His sovereignty. It was always there. We just had to receive it.

On the first Sunday in May, the worship service had gotten off to an awesome start. The presence of the Holy Spirit was definitely evident. In the congregation was a young lady who had been involved in a car accident the previous Friday night. She had attended a church conference and was en route to her home when the accident occurred. This young lady, who had been a member of my church for many years, was distraught because another driver involved in the accident had perished.

Prior to beginning his sermon, Bishop Odum asked this young lady to meet him at the altar. She was visibly shaken by what had occurred on that previous Friday night. Bishop Odum looked the young lady in the eye and explained to her that God knew her heart and knew that she would never intentionally hurt anyone. He went on to encourage her by explaining that she should not feel guilty about the accident. After speaking words of encouragement, Bishop Odum commenced to pray a fervent prayer.

Although the prayer had been specifically for the young lady at the altar, many of us listening had been moved by it. Upon completion of the heartfelt prayer, the young lady returned to her seat. She appeared to be somewhat encouraged. What we didn't realize was that this prayer was a prelude to what would transpire next.

Bishop Odum strategically scanned the congregation and fixed his eyes on a woman who had been battling cancer. He asked someone to escort her to the altar. He then turned his attention to a young man who had suffered countless bouts with sickle cell and asked his father to escort him to the altar. Each person was asked to lay prostrate before God with his or her escort kneeling. Bishop Odum continued to call names. Those called had varying afflictions, ranging from cancer to diabetes to sickle cell to heart conditions. Just about any illness one could imagine was represented on the altar that day. Regardless of the conditions, these people all had in common the fact that they were dealing with something in their bodies.

As I watched and listened, I became an army of one and began to pray silently for God's angels who were suffering. As I bowed my head and began to pray, I heard Bishop Odum's strong, authoritative voice.

"Brother Stanton, bring your wife up here. Bring Stacy up here."

Without hesitation, Jerome took me by the hand and escorted me to the altar. Enlisting the assistance of the elders and ministers of the church, Bishop Odum ensured that each person on the altar was anointed and prayed for. As he rested his hand on my forehead, I could vaguely hear Bishop Odum declaring that my womb would be opened up. He declared healing over my body and prayed for God to give Jerome the strength he needed to continue to stand with me. I truly received in my spirit everything Bishop Odum was saying because for the first time in my life, I was keenly aware of what God was capable of. As Bishop Odum and his team of elders and ministers prayed for healing all across the church, something rather profound hit me and I thought of the following passage of scripture:

And other fell on good ground, and sprang up and bear fruit an hundredfold. And when he had said these things, he cried, He that hath ears to hear, let him hear.

But that on good ground are they, which in an honest and good heart, having heard the word,
keep it, and bring forth fruit with patience. (Luke 8:8,15)

Ever since my initial miscarriage in 2002, I had been hearing the word of God. I had been instructed on how to pray with a spirit of expectancy. I had been taught to thank God for what He was *going* to do. I had heard countless sermons about faith, but it benefited me none to hear these things and not apply them to my own life. The word of God has to be planted in our spirit as a seed planted on good, fertile ground in order for it to take root and bear fruit. I finally understood this. Not only did my body have to be fertile in order for me to successfully bear a child, my spirit had to be like good ground on which the word was planted.

Knowing beyond any measure of doubt that I was in the perfect spiritual place to receive what God had in store for me, I confidently rose from my posture and returned to my seat. On the short journey to my seat, all I could do was thank God for what He was going to do in my life. Somehow, I knew it wouldn't be long. As everyone returned to their seats, Bishop Odum continued to speak declarations of healing.

As words of healing and expectancy resonated throughout the sanctuary, people were on their feet, giving God praise. It was a spirit-filled display of gratitude. As emotions ran high, a tearful Bishop Odum looked at me and boldly declared, "Stacy, you *will* have children…in the name of Jesus!" All I could do was nod. I believed what he was speaking to me. Somehow I knew that the manifestation of the blessing I so desired was on the horizon. Having heard Bishop Odum's prophetic word, I knew it wouldn't be long. God was getting ready to increase my territory, and He had allowed me to go through a mighty storm to ensure that He would get the glory and to ensure that I was prepared to fulfill the purpose He had set for my life.

Only two weeks had passed since that powerful praise and worship experience, and we were preparing to celebrate Bishop Odum's 49th birthday. To assist in this endeavor, two guest pastors were called upon to deliver the messages at 8:00a.m. and 11:00a.m., respectively. I had never heard either man preach, but I was assured they were both awesome messengers. No truer words could have been spoken.

On Sunday morning, May 21, 2006, the essence of God was seen through two of His vessels. During the 8:00a.m. worship service, we had the pleasure of hearing from Bishop Benjamin Douglas, who spoke from the subject, *The Agony of Victory*. In his own eloquent, yet dynamic manner, Bishop Douglas explained to us that we were "pregnant" with blessings, ministries, purpose, and possibilities. He went on to explain to us that in those seasons that we experience trials, Satan wants us to believe that God is aborting our blessings. In spite of Satan's intentions, it is imperative that we manifest God's presence through prayer, praise, and obedience.

I remember thinking how timely this message was. It was as though God had spoken directly into my situation. As irony would have it, Bishop Douglas had used pregnancy as his metaphor. The fecundity with which he delivered the message was riveting. I believed the message's relevance to my life was another reminder that God was about to move in a mighty way.

As if I was not already enamored by Bishop Douglas's words, the speaker for the 11:00a.m. service delivered a message I am at no risk of forgetting. His name was Bishop Darryl Woodson, and he too would prove to be a dynamic, charismatic orator. Bishop Woodson's message was titled *Don't Die in Transition*.

Bishop Woodson reminded us that there is pain associated with transition. To clarify his point, he used as his metaphor…pregnancy. Unbelievable! He explained to us that the purpose of pregnancy is not to make it to labor, but to make it to the delivery. If we give up while in labor, we will lose what God is trying to birth in us. Labor is that critical point of transition, and if we suffer through the pain associated with that transition, we will birth something beautiful. Going through labor requires patience and strength.

These messages could not have been more clear if God Himself had come down and delivered them. These men had not spoken to one another, but their sermons were amazingly similar. Their use of pregnancy as a metaphor was just so relevant to me.

As I left church that day, I thought about my situation and realized that what I had been trying to grasp for nearly four years had become crystal clear to me in a matter of four months. I had spent so much time questioning God and feeling dejected about my ongoing infertility. While I was crying, detaching myself, and experiencing feelings of inadequacy, I didn't realize that everything I needed was in the word of God. God had work for me to do, but He had to prepare me. I had been chosen to go through this storm so I would be a witness for Him, but my failure to recognize that allowed me to almost be spiritually defeated.

In the four months following my diagnosis of blocked fallopian tubes, I had conceived naturally, heard God speak to my spirit, received a prophetic word from Bishop Odum, and had that prophecy sealed by messages delivered by two ministers I had never met before. I had been in labor. I had been in transition. While I was not exactly certain when it would happen, I was certain that I was about to give birth to a miracle – spiritually and physically.

CHAPTER TWELVE

Faithful is Our God

My cup was beginning to run over! During the summer months of 2006, there was an abundance of activity to keep me busy. The interesting thing was that I was not just trying to keep busy in order to free my mind of thoughts of infertility. To say I never thought of what I had been through would be a monstrous falsity. It didn't, however, consume me the way it once did. For the first time in several years, I was living. I was simply…living.

I had put away my calendar and was no longer counting the days between menstrual cycles. I was not trying to figure out when I was ovulating. I was not having private meltdowns whenever I gave any thought to Angel or her nameless siblings. I was just living, and it was refreshing. I had put into perspective the gravity of being chosen of God for a greater purpose. I was fully aware that I was not chosen by God because I had lived a perfect, stellar life. It was by His grace. With that in mind, my grumbling and complaining had given way to humble submission and thanksgiving. What an invigorating change!

Along with twelve other candidates, Jerome and I were attending regular training sessions to prepare for the office of deacon. The more we trained, the more I realized how relevant my bout with infertility had been to this assignment, this calling. Because of my upbringing, I had always believed in God. I prayed often and sought His face in those times I felt I needed Him. However, nothing had drawn me nearer to Him than being mentally, emotionally, and spiritually broken. It was in that trustful place that I was able to humble myself and truly hear from God. It was in that place that He could use me to build up His kingdom. That's exactly where I needed to be in order to serve as deacon.

During the course of training, I came to understand that being a deacon was less about elevation and more about servitude. Being a deacon was about submission. Being a deacon was about sacrifice. I can't be certain that I would have been ready to serve in this capacity without having been broken. It was my valley experience that prepared me to heed this calling and walk in this assignment.

As we diligently studied and trained, our church began to prepare for its first annual Holy Convocation. The convocation would aptly be called *These Are They*, a title drawn from the following passage of scripture:

> *And I said unto him, Sir, thou knowest. And he said to me,*
> *These are they which came out of great tribulation,*
> *and have washed their robes, and made them white in the blood of the Lamb. (Revelation 7:14)*

Holy Convocation would commence with a service on October 15th and would culminate with a special ordination service on October 18th. It was an exciting time, to say the least. What was more exciting for me was to be sharing this experience with my husband, the very person who often prevented me from falling apart during our plight to become parents.

In addition to our rigorous training and preparation for our October ordination, Jerome and I were busy preparing for the upcoming wedding of my sister-in-law, Nicole. This was Jerome's baby sister, and we could not have been more elated for her. I was enjoying my role as matron of honor. From hosting the bridal shower to printing invitations and programs, I had made myself a committee of one to ease the bride's angst as she approached her big day.

With all that was going on, the days and weeks seemed to fly by. With the exception of the weekend that Jerome and I stole away to St. Augustine to celebrate our 6th wedding anniversary, the summer season seemed to be a blur. Before we realized it, we were traveling to South Carolina to witness my sister-in-law's nuptials. She was married in a beautiful ceremony on September 2, 2006.

Shortly after our return from Nicole's wedding, Jerome and I joined our church family in a corporate fast in preparation for Holy Convocation. During this period of fasting, I decided to spend a considerable amount of time in the word of God and in prayer. I wanted to be absolutely sure that I was ready to walk in the office of deacon. At no time did I want to take this assignment lightly.

During the first week in October, I traveled to Forsyth, GA for an operations meeting for my job. Though it was a short, overnight trip, I returned home feeling a bit under the weather. It was easy for me to attribute this to the fasting, coupled with the fact that I really needed to catch up on my rest. There I was again, feeling bad and rationalizing it. I didn't stand up and take notice until one day I felt terribly nauseated. It was not uncommon for me to experience nausea after eating something that didn't agree with me or when I became dehydrated. I just figured it was one of the two. I became a little concerned, though, when the feeling lingered for a couple of days.

One day, I was sitting at my desk completing some reports when something hit me like a ton of bricks. It was ten days into the month of October, and I had seen no signs of my menstrual cycle. I had been so busy with everything, I hadn't even noticed. Throughout my life, I had never had missed or irregular cycles, so this was definitely a sign that something was going on.

I stopped what I was doing and sat there, thinking. Nausea. Fatigue. A late menstrual period. Could it be? Could it really be? All the signs were there. The glaring, undeniable signs were there. During my lunch break, I made a quick stop by a drug store and purchased a home pregnancy test. For the remainder of the day, I could hardly concentrate on work. My mind was racing. My heart was racing. Although I said nothing to no one, something in my spirit told me it was time to start celebrating a victory.

That evening, I could not get through the door of my home fast enough. I was glad to have beaten Jerome home as I wanted to be alone when I took the test. Those had to be the longest three minutes of my life as I waited for the result to appear. I had taken countless pregnancy tests before, but this was slightly different. Jerome and I had been waiting for God to do what my doctor had said could not be done. We had stepped out on faith, probably for the first time since we began struggling with infertility. To that end, a positive outcome would speak volumes about walking in faith.

As I waited, I made a concerted effort not to look at the test. When I suspected three minutes had passed, I slowly reached for the little white stick. As I looked down at it, my heart nearly jumped out of my chest! I fixed my eyes on that little pink plus sign. Wow! A positive pregnancy test! No fertility treatments! Just faith! All I could do was go into prayer.

"Thank you, Lord! Thank you so much! Lord, I know this is the one! Thank you so much!"

I pulled myself together and began contemplating how and when I would share the news with Jerome. During the course of the week, I took four more tests. I was not taking the tests because I didn't believe the results. I think it was more about recapturing that feeling I had when I saw that little plus sign. I even took a digital test, and it clearly spelled out, "pregnant."

By Friday, I was ready to tell Jerome the good news. I had just taken the fifth pregnancy test before joining him on the couch. We engaged in small talk as he flipped through the channels on the television.

"Do you want to know what I was just doing?" I began.

"Well, I thought you were just in the bathroom."

"Oh, I was, but I need to show you something."

"Are you okay? Is something wrong?"

"Nothing's wrong, but I wanted you to see this," I said, handing him the little white stick with the digital reading.

Jerome dropped the remote control and stared at the test stick. He looked over at me with a smile and excitedly asked, "You're pregnant?"

"Yes, I'm pregnant!"

Jerome grabbed me and embraced me as if he shared my belief that this would be the one to prevail. It was amazing because neither of us appeared to have that sinking feeling we had had in the past. We were just excited!

"I haven't called Dr. Robinson yet. I'll probably do that on Monday."

"Yeah, make sure you call him *first thing* Monday morning," Jerome commanded.

On Sunday night, October 15th, Holy Convocation began. The service was awesome, and I left feeling great. What a season! This was definitely shaping up to be a great season. We were three days from becoming ordained, and I had recently learned that my season of infertility was coming to an end.

As promised, I called Dr. Robinson's office early Monday morning. Monday mornings were usually pretty hectic at work, so as soon as I was able to settle down for a moment, I called. I felt like a nervous school girl calling to ask a boy to the Sadie Hawkins dance.

"Chatham OB/GYN. May I help you?"

"Yes, I need to make an appointment with Dr. Robinson please."

"Are you a new patient?"

"No."

"Okay, what is your name, ma'am?"

"Stacy Stanton."

"Hey, Stacy! This is Sharon!"

Throughout my ordeal, I had become rather fond of Dr. Robinson's staff. These ladies were consummate professionals, much like Dr. Robinson himself. What I think will always remain indelibly imprinted in my mind will be their compassion. Although the marriage between spirituality and business was often taboo, the nurses and office staff at Chatham OB/GYN never hesitated to remind me that I was in their thoughts and prayers. They came to know me on a first-name basis and were always so polite. I could not have taken this journey with a better group of medical professionals.

"Hi, Sharon! I need to come in ASAP!"

"What's wrong, Stacy?"

"Well, I think...I am...pregnant!"

"Oh, my God, are you serious? Yeah, we need to get you in here quickly."

After reviewing Dr. Robinson's calendar, Sharon told me that he could see me on Wednesday, October 18th at 11:00a.m. As I accepted the appointment, I couldn't help thinking of the irony. That day, October 18, 2006, had been set aside as the day we would officially be ordained as deacons. Right before my eyes, everything I had been praying for was coming full circle.

I took the day off so that I could get an early start on Wednesday morning. I began my morning by getting my nails done and heading to the mall to purchase a white shirt for Jerome. As I pulled into the parking lot of the Oglethorpe Mall, my cell phone began to ring.

"Hello," I said as I pulled into a parking space designated for expectant mothers. I had to smile to myself.

"Hey, lady!" It was my friend, Kisha.

"Hey, Kish, what's going on?"

"Nothing much, girl. I just had to call and congratulate you on your ordination and to tell you I love you."

"I love you too, and thank you so much. I can't believe the day is here after all the months of training."

"I wish I could be there, but I just wanted to let you know I was thinking about you and Jerome today."

As I hung up the phone, I just sat there and smiled. What Kisha didn't know was that congratulations were in order for another reason. Jerome and I had decided to walk quietly in our blessing and be very strategic about telling our family and friends. I must admit, however, that keeping the secret was going to be painstaking at best.

As I entered the mall and began searching for Jerome's shirt, I received another phone call, this time from my friend, Lisa. She, too, was calling to congratulate me on the impending ordination. It was so nice to hear from both of these ladies. It was a small reminder of what I had learned throughout my ordeal about friendship. Going through years of infertility definitely helped me distinguish enduring friendships from fleeting ones.

With my nails done and Jerome's white shirt in hand, I headed for my car. I had about 15 minutes to make it to the doctor's office. As I pulled out of the mall parking lot, I was struck by an overwhelmingly mirthful feeling. What a beautiful day it was! Not all of my visits to Dr. Robinson's office had been marked by feelings of joy, but on this day, I couldn't get there fast enough. As I pulled into the parking lot of the Bank of America building that housed Chatham OB/GYN, my heart raced.

As I sat in the triage area, a nurse walked over and began making notes in my file. She checked my blood pressure and weight and asked me the start date of my last menstrual cycle. Too anxious to wait for her to tell me, I inquired about the results of my pregnancy test.

"Oh, it was definitely positive. You are pregnant, Stacy."

Hearing someone say it out loud made it real for me. Noticing that my blood pressure was slightly elevated, the nurse placed her hand on my shoulder and assured me that everything would be okay. She told me to calm down. Without even realizing it, I had allowed a bit of anxiety to enter my spirit. I immediately had to put that to rest. I looked at the nurse and smiled because for the first time since my miscarriage in 2002, I truly believed everything would be okay.

As I waited in the examination room for Dr. Robinson, I glanced at the calendar on his wall. I thought about how I had never been able to count past the 24th week in a pregnancy. I knew this would be different. In my heart of hearts, I just knew it. Upon entering the room, Dr. Robinson smiled and shook my hand.

"Well, how about that! Looks like we have a viable pregnancy on our hands!"

"Yes, sir, we do," I said, smiling.

"So, which treatment method did you decide on? In vitro? Insemination?"

"Well, after the consultation, I never returned to the fertility specialist. We tried something different. We tried faith."

Dr. Robinson looked excited and puzzled all at the same time. He looked back at my chart and remembered the miscarriage I had right after Easter.

"So, you have conceived twice since we diagnosed the blocked tubes. How about that."

I could tell that Dr. Robinson was amazed by what God had done. I told him that Jerome and I decided to believe in God's promise and just wait. He nodded almost in agreement. I say almost in agreement because I knew he was trying to keep it strictly professional and avoid a religious exchange with me. Not much needed to be said, though, because we knew what the laparoscopy had revealed. We further knew what had transpired since the procedure. Any reasonable person could have drawn whatever inference he wished, but I knew who had made this possible.

Dr. Robinson administered an ultrasound and was able to locate the amniotic sack. He then began the task of mapping out plans for the pregnancy.

"Based on your last menstrual cycle, we have a due date of June 13th. What I would like to do is place a cerclage in December."

Dr. Robinson went on to explain to me that he would be sending me to Savannah Perinatology, so the cerclage could be placed by a specialist. I was immediately started on progesterone and prenatal vitamins. I knew I was in good hands as Dr. Robinson had followed my case from the very beginning.

I was completely enamored by God and what He was doing in my life. Just nine months prior, I had received pictures of my blocked fallopian tubes. Just look at what mustard seed faith had done for Jerome and me!

*   *   *

The procession was beautiful. The music was serene, but spirit-filled. The ordination service was awesome and spiritually charged. As the final night of an awesome Holy Convocation, it was destined to be an unforgettable night. In addition to the 14 candidates for the office of deacon, there were five candidates to be ordained as elders.

In spite of the anointed music, the beautiful procession of candidates, the sea of worshippers that filled the sanctuary, and the presence of the Holy Spirit, the most abiding memory would lie in the words spoken by Bishop Odum. While he acknowledged that there was cause for celebration, he wanted to impress upon us the gravity of being called to serve as officers in the Lord's house.

Using the vivid metaphor of dawn, Bishop painted a poignant picture for us about the time of preparation. His message was that in order for us to be fully prepared for the work we must do in the day, we had to get up at dawn. He recalled his mother getting up at dawn to prepare breakfast when he was just a boy. He made reference to fishermen getting up at dawn to catch the fish while they were biting.

At dawn, three things needed to happen. We needed to wake up, wash up, and dress up. Waking up involved our alertness. Washing up involved spiritual cleansing, and dressing up involved putting on our commitment, our battle dress, and our desire to please God. It was a candid message of admonishment. It was a call to action. It was a grave reminder of the seriousness of this undertaking.

On that night, Bishop Odum laid hands on Jerome, me, and 12 other men and women, ordaining us to the office of deacon. On that night, our lives changed, not only because we had become deacons, but because we were carrying tangible evidence of God's power and His faithfulness. On that night, we were ordained deacons and parents!

CHAPTER THIRTEEN

The Perfect Pregnancy

My pregnancy coordinator. That is how Dr. Robinson described himself. He would take a proactive approach to ensuring the success of my pregnancy. His philosophy was that while we could not control the outcome, we could do everything within our power to try and secure a positive one. This was extremely reassuring for me because even with my faith building, my history with early pregnancy loss made it somewhat difficult to just relax and enjoy this nine-month ride.

I can vividly recall a cold morning in November. Because of my mother's work schedule, I had been tasked with getting my brother and nephew to school. It was a beautiful, peaceful morning, but there was a sharpness about the cold that was not characteristic of the Savannah area. I had grown so accustomed to morning sickness that I had built an immeasurable tolerance for the constant nausea. Because of that, it rarely interfered with my daily living activities.

On this cold morning, however, I felt discomfort that went beyond morning sickness. What I felt could easily be likened to a dull, constant menstrual cramp. While I was reluctant to panic, I felt this pain warranted some attention. Relieved to have made it safely to the boys' school, I dropped them off and pulled into the parking lot so I could call Dr. Robinson's office. When Sharon answered the phone, I explained to her what I was feeling.

"Stacy, you need to be on your way! You know Dr. Robinson doesn't play when it comes to you!"

I could not help but chuckle when I thought of how protective the staff was of this pregnancy. Not wanting to take any chances that something might go wrong, I headed right over. After a thorough ultrasound and a check of my cervix, I was assured that everything looked great. What Dr. Robinson did find was a couple of cervical polyps. While they could cause some mild discomfort, I was assured they should not adversely impact my pregnancy.

"I'll be glad when we make it to December," Dr. Robinson said, looking at the calendar on the wall.

My appointment with Savannah Perinatology had already been set, and we were just waiting it out. Each passing day and each passing week represented a small victory. It was nearly impossible for me to avoid being consumed by this pregnancy, and I would often sit and daydream about my baby being here. With the excitement surrounding the pregnancy, Jerome and I found it increasingly difficult to keep it a secret. While Jerome's best friend, Tony, and his wife were visiting with us, Jerome disclosed the pregnancy. They were both very excited for us. We also decided to tell our mothers and sisters, who all seemed to be overjoyed by the news.

Jerome and I prayed daily for the health of the baby growing inside of me. I even prayed that God would help me to avoid waking up each morning wondering if *that* would be the day something went wrong. That kind of thinking would definitely make for a long journey to my due date.

As December approached, I looked forward to having my cerclage placed. I think Dr. Robinson, Jerome, and I were kind of holding our breaths awaiting this milestone in the pregnancy. Because of my unfortunate history, I was a little surprised by what happened when I visited Savannah Perinatology. This is how I pictured it. I would have a routine ultrasound, and my surgery would likely be scheduled for the following week. I had even alerted my supervisor that I would probably be out for about a week in December due to a minor surgery. What I had pictured was not at all what happened.

One of the perinatologists administered an abdominal and transvaginal ultrasound just as I had expected. However, what happened next was rather puzzling. The perinatologist, referencing my ultrasound image on a computer monitor, showed me that my cervix was measuring very long and closed shut.

"So, what does this mean in terms of the cerclage placement?" I asked.

"Mrs. Stanton, I have reviewed your record, and I do understand Dr. Robinson's concerns, but at this juncture, we cannot justify placing a cerclage."

My heart began to race as I processed what the doctor was telling me. Although I was elated that my cervix was in great shape, I felt a little uneasy about going through the pregnancy without a cerclage. The doctor, whose demeanor was much more pleasant than that of the fertility specialist I had visited, went on to tell me that he wanted to see me again in two weeks. If there were any changes in the length of my cervix, they would proceed with the surgery to place the cerclage.

As soon as I left Savannah Perinatology, I phoned Dr. Robinson, who was not at all pleased with the outcome of my appointment. Whether my cervix appeared to be closed or not, he wanted the cerclage in place before any trouble arose. While I agreed with his logic, I felt this was God's subtle way of reminding me that when He was ready to move in my situation, He was not going to *partially* move. It was going to be all or nothing. Either I was going to be completely healed or not healed at all. After all, the God who released the blockages in my fallopian tubes could certainly hold my cervix in place.

During that two-week period that I awaited my second appointment with Savannah Perinatology, I contacted my best friend, Stephanie, and asked if I could treat her to lunch for her birthday. During our outing, I shared with her our great news. Before I could get all the words out, she began smiling and stated that she could not have asked for a better birthday present. Stephanie told me that she wanted to help host my baby shower, something I had not even thought about. I nodded because in my heart, I knew we'd make to that point in the pregnancy this time. Satan would have had me doubt this, but I was not going to ruin this pregnancy by not believing.

Approximately one week after my lunch outing with Stephanie, I arrived for my second appointment at Savannah Perinatology. I wasn't sure what to expect, but I was prepared. I knew that I would either be scheduling my surgery or reporting back to Dr. Robinson that there would be no surgery.

"Your cervix is still long," the doctor said, pointing at the computer monitor, "I just don't see a need to place a cerclage at this time."

The doctor went on to point out the risks involved in having a cerclage placed. One risk, which I had learned during my pregnancy with Angel, was the premature rupture of membranes. He felt that if the cervix was holding, it would not be logical to place a cerclage and risk sending me into premature labor.

Once again, I left Savannah Perinatology with a report that my cervix was showing no signs of opening up. Once again, I left without scheduling surgery. After my second visit with Savannah Perinatology, Dr. Robinson scheduled an appointment with Jerome and me to discuss our options. He informed us that although he wanted the cerclage placed by the specialists at Savannah Perinatology, he could do it himself if necessary. The other option would be to just monitor the pregnancy very closely and be prepared to respond to any changes in my cervix. True to form, Jerome and I had to ask the glaring question.

"What has been your experience with high-risk pregnancies where cerclages were not placed?" I asked.

"Well," Dr. Robinson began, "I have to be honest with you. I have seen it go both ways. I've seen situations similar to yours where there was no cerclage placed, and the pregnancies ensued without any problems. Unfortunately, I have also had patients who opted not to have the cerclages placed, and the pregnancies were not sustained."

He went on to explain that a cerclage does not guarantee that there will be no complications during the pregnancy. Of course, my pregnancy with Angel was evidence of that. After much careful thought, Jerome and I decided to forego the surgery. Some would be reluctant to agree with that decision, but we realized that not everyone knew what we knew about how this pregnancy would end.

With the issue of the cerclage behind us, we proceeded with weekly visits to Chatham OB/GYN. Before I even realized it, I was in my second trimester and had begun to develop the proverbial baby bump. To those who saw me frequently, pregnancy was beginning to be obvious. Some people even asked me outright if I was, in fact, pregnant. Notwithstanding the inappropriateness of such question, I was somewhat flattered that I was starting to visibly wear my little miracle.

This pregnancy became more and more real to us each day. Every appointment was a reminder that this was a strong, healthy pregnancy. Our baby's heartbeat was as vibrant as ever, and he was developing at a normal rate. Yes, we had even learned, almost accidentally, that we were having a boy. During one of my routine ultrasounds, the technician excitedly blurted out the baby's gender without asking if we wanted to know. We were too excited to be angry with her.

During the month of January, my mother secured the Eden Room at my church as the venue for the baby shower. Helping her host the shower would be Yashica, Stephanie, and my sister-in-law, Nicole. It seemed surreal to be at that point in the pregnancy where plans for the shower were beginning. This pregnancy was real! The pregnancy that was not supposed to occur without fertility treatments was undoubtedly real!

As the morning sickness tapered off, I found that I was sleeping less and feeling much better. Each day was as fresh as the morning dew. After three miscarriages and a premature delivery, I was finally learning what it was like to experience a viable pregnancy, and I wanted to soak in every moment. Those who knew of the pregnancy at this juncture ensured us they would pray without ceasing. Our family and friends, including our church family, rallied around Jerome and me with undying support. I was certain that the love and support surrounding us could be felt by our baby.

Dr. Robinson was pleased with the progress of the pregnancy and set as our next major milestone, Easter. Easter would mark the 30th week of my pregnancy. Dr. Robinson indicated to us that once we reached 30 weeks' gestation, we would be on the home stretch. He felt confident that once we reached 30 weeks, even if the baby was born, we should be okay.

To commemorate Angel's birthday in March, Jerome and I set aside that day to set up our first baby registry. Instead of setting the registry up online, we decided to actually go into the store so we could scan the items we wanted. This was the first time since Angel's death that we could make a happy memory on her birthday. As was true of each of Angel's birthdays, I received phone calls from Kisha and Lisa. What these ladies didn't know, though, was that I had quite a surprise in store for them.

As time marched on, I began to grow weary of the frequent doctor's visits and ultrasounds, but I understood the rationale. Some visits would consist only of a brief exchange whereby Dr. Robinson asked how I was feeling and if I had any questions. The routine had become mundane, but I refused to miss an appointment. I knew that getting our little miracle to the finish line had to be a team effort.

The further we progressed in the pregnancy, the more discussions we began to have about the delivery. Although I would have preferred a vaginal delivery, Dr. Robinson felt it would be too risky. Having undergone two major abdominal surgeries, I was at risk of suffering uterine rupture during delivery. Dr. Robinson explained to me that even if I went into labor, he would perform a cesarean section. Risking uterine rupture would negate all of our efforts. While I was okay with the decision to have a cesarean delivery, I was a little uneasy because of the unbearable pain I endured after Angel's birth. I could recall barely being able to walk, but I resolved that my pain was a small price to pay for my baby's safe delivery.

Before we realized it, Jerome and I were in church, celebrating the resurrection of our Lord and Savior, Jesus Christ. Easter Sunday had arrived, and I was 30.5 weeks pregnant! No cerclage. No changes in my cervix. No spotting. No more cramping. This was shaping up to be the perfect pregnancy by all accounts. By this time, we had shared our news with everyone, even our family and friends who were out of town. Everyone we knew was witnessing the miracle that was unfolding right before our eyes.

With only three weeks to go, plans for our unisex baby shower had nearly wrapped. Everything was in place, and it was only a matter of tying a few loose ends. This was all so surreal, and I couldn't help thinking about how God had moved. He had allowed us to go through a major storm in order to strengthen our faith and prepare us for the work He had in store for us. He moved in His own time and healed my body in such a way that only He could get the glory.

This pregnancy was very real, but as real as it was, so was the tumultuous journey we took through infertility. Even in rejoicing, I couldn't forget what I had been brought through. Contrary to what my prognosis indicated, I conceived naturally and was carrying a baby boy, a beautiful, healthy baby boy!

CHAPTER FOURTEEN

The Manifestation

The sun shone brightly, and there was no cloud in sight. It was the most beautiful of days, and my heart was filled with joy. Overcome with excitement, I had awakened early. After months of planning, the day had arrived for our baby shower. Ironically, it was also the day for the annual March of Dimes walk. It was April 28, 2007, and nothing could steal my joy.

Although the Earth Angels Family Team participated in the walk, Jerome and I decided that I should forego the event. This decision came on the heels of an impromptu nosebleed the night before. Jerome implored me to stay home and rest while he and several of our friends attended the walk. Because of my pregnancy, I had not given WalkAmerica the time and attention I had in the previous two years. That didn't stop us, however, from receiving the honor of Top Family Team for the third consecutive year. Although I could not physically be there, I was so proud to be a part of this endeavor.

We had several friends and family members who had traveled to be with us on our special day. Among those were our own houseguests, which included my friend, Lisa, and her family and my sister-in-law, Nicole, and her family. As Nicole spent the day running errands with Yashica, Lisa and I spent some quiet time at my home. We reflected, laughed, cried, laughed some more, reflected some more, and just basked in the miracle that was unfolding before us. This was like a dream. Having passed all the milestones Dr. Robinson set, I was 33.5 weeks into my pregnancy.

I was well aware of the work that had gone into planning the baby shower, but nothing could have prepared me for what I would see upon walking into the Eden Room. It was beautifully decorated with blue and yellow balloons, table cloths, and centerpieces. The room held the aroma of deliciously prepared food. As guests began to arrive, our gift table began to fill up with just about any baby necessity one could imagine. This display nearly brought me to tears. As I perused the room, I thought of all the prayer warriors who had been interceding on our behalf.

Jerome and I were thrown a baby shower that would rival some wedding receptions. My mom, Stephanie, Yashica, and Nicole truly did an awesome job. The shower was complete with an opening prayer by Bishop Odum, remarks by our First Lady, Sheila Odum, solos, poetry, games, food and door prizes. With the help of my friend, Karen, I was even able to deliver a slide presentation that told the story of our testimony. I wanted to share our story in this manner because most people in the room were only aware of parts of the testimony. For the first time, everyone heard *everything* we had experienced, and we were hard pressed to find a dry eye in the room.

As I glanced about the room, I could not help thinking of the conversations I had had with several of the people about my infertility. I could not help thinking how so any people had encouraged me. There were people who actually believed all along that God would bless Jerome and me according to the desires of our hearts. Our guests had come from all over – Columbia, SC, Clio, SC, Charlotte, NC, Atlanta, GA, Swainsboro, GA, and Albany, GA. Regardless of the origin, none of these angels thought it was robbery of their time for them to be with us that day.

As Yashica gave her remarks, she spoke publicly for the first time about her experience with ovarian cancer. My mother followed with her declaration that God had healed both her daughters. Our baby shower had served as a platform to remind people of the true goodness of God, and my heart was so full.

Later that evening as I perused the guest book, I realized that 108 guests had attended our celebration. This number was definitely reflected in the myriad of gifts we received. Even with all the gifts that had been given to us, I was more enamored by the spiritual manifestation of love.

During the week following the baby shower, I spent much of my time opening gifts, writing thank-you cards, and organizing the nursery. I would spend a few moments each day standing over the crib, imagining my baby lying there. We were only 5 ½ weeks from his delivery, and he had become even more real to me. He was so active in my womb, a clear sign that he was healthy.

Still concerned about uterine rupture, Dr. Robinson made the decision to deliver the baby one week prior to my due date. This was in hopes that I would not go into labor. That was great for me because the sooner we could see our little boy, the better. I was also happy about this because of the physical changes in my body during the final stages of the pregnancy. My feet were terribly swollen, and getting comfortable in bed was nearly impossible. To me, these were small prices to pay for the gift God had bestowed upon Jerome and me.

My last day at work was May 25, 2007. I decided to allow myself two weeks to rest and prepare for the delivery. I also had to consider the possibility that I could go into labor prior to my due date. My days were spent lounging on my mother's couch while Jerome was at work. Because I live outside of Savannah, my mother was concerned about me being at home alone and possibly going into labor. I thought it was so sweet how protective she still was of Yashica and me despite the fact that we were adults. Each day was a new adventure. Although our baby shower was over, there was a package waiting on our porch nearly every day during the weeks that followed.

Jerome and I started every morning with a prayer for our son's safe delivery. Remembering my near-death experience with Angel, Jerome also prayed for me to be okay during the birth. During this time, I could not help recalling Bishop Woodson's message, *Don't Die in Transition*. We had not endured five years of infertility only to get this close and face a tragedy. God had not brought us this far to leave us now. He had done what was not believed possible through carnal eyes. It was only a matter of bringing forth the fruit.

Our doorbell rang at approximately 2:00a.m. on Wednesday, June 6, 2007. It was Yashica, who had driven from Atlanta to witness the birth of her nephew. This birth would represent so many things for our family. Having endured so much longsuffering, we were reminded that even in times of trouble, the perfect will of God would prevail. I was grateful that Yashica was able to share this occasion with us. She had been through her own health crisis, but God is truly a healer.

At approximately 6:35a.m., Jerome and I arrived at Memorial Health University Medical Center. Without delay, the staff began prepping me for my cesarean delivery. I was given a hospital gown and a bag for my clothes. Once I was all changed into the gown, I was connected to a machine that would monitor the baby's heartbeat. My palms were pouring with sweat. When I was being prepped for Angel's delivery, it seemed like a nightmare, but this, more like a fairytale. This was finally going to happen. The baby's heart sounded stronger than ever.

For a brief moment, I felt a slight heaviness in my heart for Angel. How could I not think of her? She had been born in this very hospital, via the same method, possibly in the same room. Three years had passed, but I knew undoubtedly that she would always be in my heart.

After four attempts, my IV was placed, and at that juncture, Jerome and I received a detailed explanation of what would transpire. I would be given an epidural, and barring any complications with that, Jerome would be escorted into the room to accompany me for the procedure. If complications did arise during the administering of the epidural, I would be put to sleep, and Jerome would not be allowed in the room. It was also explained to us that the condition of the baby at birth would determine what happened next. If the baby was in distress, he would be taken to the NICU, but if he is breathing on his own and responding well, he might be able to join me in recovery. While I knew the nursing staff had to explain everything to us in great detail, I completely brushed off the last statement. You see, I knew that when God moved, He moved. There we were, in the hospital, just moments from seeing the physical manifestation of a miracle. In distress? No, not *this* child. His destiny was already written.

Soon after we received our marching orders, Dr. Robinson walked in the room appearing to be very jovial.

"Is this the Stanton residence?" he asked jokingly.

We all laughed. The mood about the room was cheerful as we all realized that this was the first time the Stanton's had a pregnancy ending on a high note. I finally knew what my friends, my sister, and every woman who had birthed a child had felt. Even before the physical birth, the maternal instinct kicks in. The desire to protect becomes strong. It is like no other feeling in the world.

Dr. Robinson chatted with us a bit, checked the monitor and explained that he would see us in the operating room. I was then introduced to the person who would be my best friend throughout the procedure, my anesthesiologist. I received the standard speech about the risks of anesthesiology and what I could expect from my epidural.

Before I realized it, I was being wheeled back. I glanced over at Jerome, who would wait to be called back. He nodded at me, and I smiled at him. I felt a little strange going back without him. I wanted him next to me every second, but I had to be a big girl. This was what I had been praying for, so I needed to be ready to receive it.

As I was being wheeled back, I became extremely cold and was immediately covered with a warm blanket. With each step, my heart raced a little more. Before long, we were going through the double doors into the operating room. As I entered the room, I managed to look around. There seemed to be so many people there, and they were all preparing for the birth of *my* baby. The surgical technician was preparing the instruments. The NICU staff was on hand. The scale was ready. Everyone was ready and waiting…for *my* baby! The time had come.

With the exception of an onset of nausea, my epidural was administered with no complications, and Jerome was escorted in to join me. Shortly after his arrival, the sheet went up to block my view of the procedure. This was it! With Jerome on my right and my anesthesiologist on my left, I was alerted that the procedure was beginning. Once Dr. Robinson announced that he was beginning, he didn't say anything else to me. He spoke only to his medical staff. All I could do was lay there and wait. Jerome was holding my hand. He occasionally peeked over the sheet as I stared at the ceiling. After several minutes, I heard something very exciting. For the first time since the procedure began, Dr. Robinson spoke to me.

"Three-minute warning, Stacy! We're about to have a baby!"

I experienced this strange combination of excitement and anxiety. We were actually minutes away from the greatest breakthrough in my life. A tear rolled down my face, and Jerome gently wiped it. I maintained a tight grip on his hand, and within moments, I felt it! I felt pressure in my abdominal area that almost made me jump from the table, and then…

"Hey, how about that! He's a fine boy!"

As I heard my baby's strong, steady cry, I could hear movement across the room. The anesthesiologist placed his hand on my shoulder and congratulated me. Jerome and I smiled at each other like we had just won the lottery. We listened to everything that was going on around us as Dr. Robinson worked at closing my incision.

"Time of birth, 7:56a.m.!"

"Congratulations, Mr. and Mrs. Stanton!"

"Weight - 7 pounds, 14 ounces!"

"Length – 20 inches!"

"Agar – 9!"

"Come on over, Dad! Get some pictures!"

As I was wheeled to the recovery room, Jerome retreated to the waiting room to inform my mother and Yashica that our little man was here. My healthy baby boy was able to join me in the recovery room. I could not stop crying. He was absolutely gorgeous! He was perfect! He was mine! He was really mine! After a five-year bout with infertility, a faltering faith, a growing faith, five surgeries, and a grim prognosis, it was over. God had shown that all we have to do is trust His plan for our lives. Had that baby I was carrying in 2002 survived, would I have fully appreciated the blessing? Maybe I would have, but having gone through this journey, there is absolutely no question of who gets the glory!

We were honored with the task of naming our son, and we wanted a name that would be appropriate. In thinking on his name, we thought of how Moses was commanded by God to send some of the leaders of the Israelites to explore the land of Canaan, which God was giving to them. Moses sent the men to see if the land was fertile, whether the people who dwelled therein were strong or weak, and what kind of towns they lived in. He also told the men to bring back some of the fruit of the land. Upon returning to Moses, the men presented a cluster of grapes they had retrieved and reported that the land flowed with milk and honey. They also reported that those who dwelled in the land of Canaan were powerful and lived in large, fortified cities. Their account was that the land could not be overtaken because the dwellers were stronger than they were and that the land devours its inhabitants.

The men were silenced by Caleb, son of Jephunneh, as we are told in the following passage of scripture:

And Caleb stilled the people before Moses, and said, Let us go up at once, and possess it; for we are well able to overcome it. (Numbers 13:30)

Much like Caleb, our son would exude strength in the wake of adversity. He would be powerful, faithful, and determined. With that in mind, we chose as our son's name *Caleb Jerome Stanton*. We would work to ensure that he reverently feared God and that he understood that he could achieve anything with God by his side. On June 6, 2007 at 7:56a.m., God manifested the miraculous harvest of our seeds of faith, seeds that had to be planted in a place of brokenness. He did what man thought was not possible, and He did it in such a way that only He could be glorified. He even allowed my sister, who had battled ovarian cancer, to be there to witness it. That day became our someday, and we praise Him for the miracle…everyday!

Epilogue

We are never really sure how God will move in our lives. When I set about the task of becoming a mother, I had no idea the journey would bring so much pain and heartache to my life and the life of my husband. There was a point where we didn't believe this would ever happen for us. One day, God began to speak to our spirits about what He required of us. When we started to pray and search the scriptures, we realized that it would take a move in our faith walk for God to move in our situation. The Bible tells us that unto whomsoever much is given, of him shall much be required. (Luke 12:48)

We were never promised an easy ride. We were never promised there would not be trials. What we were promised was that God would give us strength to endure. All we have to do is trust Him. We realize that as long as we live, we will experience other trials, but it is our belief that this valley experience better equipped us to weather the storms of life.

Your storm may not be a storm of infertility. You may have a different cross to bear, but what should hold true should be your undying faith in the promise of God. Be willing to listen to that quiet, still voice. Be willing to go through your storms. Be willing to rejoice with those who rejoice and weep with those who weep. Most of all, be willing to be broken. It is on the good, fertile ground of brokenness that seeds of belief are planted and miraculous fruit is harvested!

LaVergne, TN USA
16 July 2010
189777LV00004B/12/P